The Juice Lady's

SUGAR
KNOCKOUT

D0963588

The Juice Lady's

SUGAR
KNOCKOUT

CHERIE CALBOM, MS, CN

SILOAM

Most CHARISMA HOUSE BOOK GROUP products are available at special quantity discounts for bulk purchase for sales promotions, premiums, fundraising, and educational needs. For details, write Charisma House Book Group, 600 Rinehart Road, Lake Mary, Florida 32746, or telephone (407) 333-0600.

THE JUICE LADY'S SUGAR KNOCKOUT by Cherie Calbom
Published by Siloam
Charisma Media/Charisma House Book Group
600 Rinehart Road
Lake Mary, Florida 32746
www.charismahouse.com

Cover design by Justin Evans

Visit the author's website at www.juiceladycherie.com.

Library of Congress Cataloging-in-Publication Data:
An application to register this book for cataloging has been submitted to the Library of Congress.
International Standard Book Number: 978-1-62998-722-4
E-book ISBN: 978-1-62998-723-1

First edition

16 17 18 19 20 — 987654321
Printed in the United States of America

CONTENTS

IT'S TIME TO KNOCK OUT
THAT SWEET TOOTH!

HAVE YOU BEEN thinking you need to do something about your sweet tooth and those fattening little calories that catch you off guard? Maybe you're just wanting to make a few changes when it comes to sugar. Perhaps you know you have a full-blown addiction to sweets, or maybe you are not convinced you need to make any changes at all.

Wherever you are on the spectrum, I hope my book compels you to get rid of sugar for good. I know that may sound scary, that you might never be able to enjoy a sweet treat again, but don't worry. You will still have plenty of options for sweets that are healthier for you. I have a whole dessert chapter made with healthy sweeteners.

The heart of the matter is that sugar is in almost all packaged foods today, and it's killing us slowly, while addicting us and causing us to want more and more. It did that to me. Sugar ruined my health and nearly destroyed my life. I believe it was a big part of killing my mother with cancer early in life. She loved sweets and didn't like vegetables; cancer cells use sugar for fuel (glycolytic fermentation). I'll tell you more about that later. Right now, I want you to know that science supports what I say and what I experienced.

The Journal of Neuroscience and Biobehavioral Reviews (2008) looked at sugar and how addictive it can be. This research involved rats because they can become addicted to abusive drugs in a similar manner to human beings. This study indicated that in certain circumstances, "access to sugar can lead to behavioral and neurochemical changes that resemble the effects of substance abuse."[1] The evidence showed clearly: sugar is addictive! Scientists said this study proved what was already known: sugar affects the same neural pathways as illegal drugs. We get hooked because sugar gives us pleasure. But why does it give us so much pleasure? A study published in 2002 by the North American Association for the Study of Obesity showed that sugar produces a release of dopamine and opiates in the nucleus accumbens, which is the reward system of the brain.[2] And listen up! This is the same area of the brain that drugs like nicotine and cocaine stimulate.

Not everyone is addicted to sugar, but almost everyone eats too much of this stuff because food manufacturers put it in nearly everything. We've gotten used to a sweeter taste, so food producers are even putting sweetener in many food products that formerly never contained sweetener, like lunch meats and almond butter. Certain people have a predisposition to sugar stimulation; it can cause a full-blown addiction in these individuals. They develop overwhelming cravings. Even in the face of negative physical consequences, such as weight gain, diabetes, or hypoglycemia, they are unable to quit or even reduce their intake. They are sugar addicts.

But here's the good news: Sugar addiction *can* be beaten. I overcame a powerful sugar addition, and you can too. You must want this sincerely. You must work at it fervently. If you are addicted, you can be free of sugar's lure. That's what this book is all about—helping you knock sugar out of your life. You can overcome the power of this reward-seeking behavior and not want sugar ever again. Let me tell you my story.

My Bout With Sugar Addiction

I was totally addicted to sugar as a child. It is said that on an emotional level a craving for sweets can be prompted by the need to bring more sweetness into one's life. That was true for me, having lost my mother at age six to breast cancer. But there was something else going on as well. I was addicted to the chemistry of sugar. It engaged the pleasure center of my brain, and there were times when I just couldn't stop eating it.

I remember one day after a wedding at the church where my aunt and uncle pastored that I pulled the cake box out of the garbage and polished off all the leftover cake and frosting. I was only fifteen, but even then I knew something was really wrong.

Throughout my whole childhood, I was nearly always sick with colds or the flu. I rarely remember feeling great, and sometimes I felt worse than others. I have many memories of eating sweets, such as ice cream shakes my dad made with old-fashioned malted milk, cinnamon rolls my grandmother baked with love and oodles of frosting, and loads of candy, cookies, cakes, and anything else sweet I could find. I'd eat sweets until I felt as if I were nearly in a trance. Once I started, I couldn't stop until the carton, bag, batch, or whatever I had was gone.

I remember being foggy-brained even as a child. In high school, one of my teachers called me his favorite roller coaster student because my grades were up and down, my brain on and off, depending probably on how much sugar I'd eaten and how much it had spaced out my mind.

I struggled on through my twenties until I got so sick I could no longer work. I had to quit my job as I turned thirty. And it was a fun job. I worked for Pat Boone in Hollywood and was having a "gee-I'm-not-in-Kansas-anymore" kind of time, meeting many interesting people like Kathie Lee Gifford (she wasn't Gifford then). In fact we had a double date to the first Star Wars movie. But right in the middle of an interesting life, I developed a severe case of chronic fatigue syndrome and fibromyalgia that made me so sick I couldn't work any longer. I felt as though I had a never-ending flu. I was lethargic and constantly feverish with swollen glands. I was in non-stop pain. My body ached all over.

I had to move back to my father's home in Colorado to try to recover. But recovery didn't come with a prescription pad. Not one doctor could tell me what I should do to improve my health. One said I might be depressed. No, I had been having the time of my life until I got sick. I realized I needed to do my own research and decided that everything I had been eating was tearing down my health rather than healing my body. I didn't like vegetables. I loved junk food, fast food, and, of course, sweets. Because of my research, I started to call sugar "demon sugar," and out it went from my life.

When I read about juicing and whole foods, it made sense. So I bought a juicer and designed a program I could follow. I began my health regimen with a five-day vegetable juice fast. Then I continued juicing and eating whole foods for three months. I cut out all sweets. I ate strictly, never cheating once. I was so desperate to win this fight for my health.

One morning I woke up around 8:00 a.m., which was early for me then, without an alarm sounding off. I felt as if someone had given me a new body in the night. I had so much energy that I actually wanted to exercise. What had happened? This new feeling of good health and vitality had just appeared with the morning sun. But my body had been healing all along; it just had not manifested fully until that day. I felt such a wonderful sense of being alive! I looked and felt completely renewed.

After my own experience, receiving a graduate degree in whole foods nutrition, all the people I've worked with, and the research I've done, I'm convinced that sugar is at the root of many health challenges. If you're struggling with your health, healing can happen for you too. There is hope, no matter what health challenges you face. But one thing I know: whether it is foggy brain, fatigue, or more serious health problems like cancer, the first place you need to start is rooting sugar out of your diet. In fact, if you came to me for nutrition counseling, and you asked what single behavior would have the greatest effect in turning your health around, I would tell you to cut out sweets. Start there, and it will have a huge impact on your health. Then, of course, start juicing vegetables.

Sugar Punch

My hope is that this book will truly inspire you to knock sugar out of your life for good so that you will experience firsthand the healing, rejuvenating power of a sugar-free life. I chose the "knock out" theme because it's been a winner when it came to saturated animal fat. I was a spokesperson for the *Lean, Mean, Fat-Reducing Grilling Machine*. I also wrote *Knock-Out-the-Fat Barbecue and Grilling Cookbook* with George Foreman. I appeared in several infomercials with George and on QVC with the grills for over thirteen years. That was one of the most successful campaigns in the history of the western world. The product was good and the education was very helpful. But if I could have found a product that would have knocked out sugar like we knocked out fat, the health of a huge number of Americans would have improved dramatically.

Now I have a product to help you knock out sugar: this book. The "knock out" theme runs throughout the pages that follow. If you're unconvinced that sweets could be responsible for any ailments, I've included scores of scientific journal references that will hopefully convince you that there is merit to my premise. If you want to get off sweets but don't know how to escape the clutches of the sugar trap, I have a program that can help you kick the habit for good.

Years ago, when I first met George in Las Vegas where he was fighting and I was demonstrating a Juiceman juicer for Salton Housewares, he gave me two little red boxing gloves on a key chain with an autographed photo. They hung on a bulletin board in my office for years, a reminder that we can knock unwanted foods and substances out of our diets and out of our lives for good. We can live life as winners! You can be sugar free and healthy with plenty of energy to win the fights of your life.

I hope you enjoy reading *The Juice Lady's Sugar Knockout*. And whether you have diabetes, hypoglycemia, heart problems, fatigue, foggy brain, or just a feeling of malaise, or sub-optimal health, or you want to lose weight, it is my prayer that this book will help you find your path to vibrant health.

Chapter 1

SUGAR'S LOW BLOW TO OUR HEALTH AND WELLNESS

THERE IS A criminal in our pantries stealing our health, wealth, and happiness and causing us to gain weight. It's well disguised and "getting away with murder," as they say. Almost everyone loves it, but it should be tried for crimes against humanity. Its name? Sugar.

What sweet treat traps you in its lair? Chocolates, fancy cupcakes with swirling frosting, or colorful scoops of ice cream? They all appear so attractive and taste really delicious. All seems well until sugar has you cornered in its den. "Villain in Disguise?" asked a headline in a 1977 issue of the *New York Times*. We ask today, "Is sugar actually toxic?"

Conventional wisdom has long said that at its worst, sugar only causes tooth decay and makes us fat due to the empty calories we consume in excess because it tastes so good. Is this wisdom or a sweet lullaby lie?

Sugar does more than make us fat; it makes us sick too. "Sugar has unique characteristics, specifically in the way the human body metabolizes the fructose in it," says Robert Lustig, a specialist of pediatric hormone disorders and the leading expert in childhood obesity at the University of California, San Francisco, School of Medicine.[1] Lustig is famous for his viral YouTube video "Sugar:

The Bitter Truth." Sugar, he says, is "singularly harmful."[2] What about singularly toxic?

If you're leaning toward believing that sugar is toxic, you're not alone. Lustig says sugar is a toxic substance that people abuse. In Lustig's view, we should see sugar that same way we see cigarettes—as a toxic substance that is killing us.[3]

New York Times writer Gary Taubes says, "to claim that one particularly cherished aspect of our diet might not just be an unhealthful indulgence but actually be toxic, that when you bake your children a birthday cake or give them lemonade on a hot summer day, you may be doing them more harm than good, despite all the love that goes with it. Suggesting that sugar might kill us is what zealots do. But Lustig, who has genuine expertise, has accumulated and synthesized a mass of evidence, which he finds compelling enough to convict sugar."[4]

Journalists such as Gary Taubes and Mark Bittman have found in their research that sugar harms our body's organs and also disrupts our hormonal cycles. They say that consuming sugar in excess is a primary cause of obesity and metabolic disorders such as diabetes and cardiovascular disease. According to the Centers for Disease Control, more than one-third of adults and approximately 12.7 million children and adolescents in the United States are obese.[5] And the CDC also reports that 29.1 million Americans have diabetes. That's 9.3 percent of the US population.[6] But that's not all. Many people are affected by ailments and annoyances such as insomnia, colds, flu, skin problems, an impaired immune system, fatigue, sinus problems, and headaches. Over and over in my nutritional practice, I've seen such maladies link back to sugar, and when my clients stopped eating it, the symptoms went away.

What Makes Sugar a Toxic Contender?

The words *toxicity* and *detox* are very popular today. Most people will say they feel toxic from time to time. But what is toxicity as it relates to the human body? Harrison's *Principles of Internal Medicine* says toxicity is "the degree to which a substance can harm humans or animals." It further states:

> Acute toxicity involves harmful effects in an organism through a single or short-term exposure. Subchronic toxicity is the ability of a toxic substance to cause effects for more than one year but less than the lifetime of the exposed organism. Chronic toxicity is the ability of a substance or mixture of substances to cause harmful effects over an extended period, usually upon repeated or continuous exposure, sometimes lasting for the entire life of the exposed organism.[7]

Gary Taubes writes, "As Lustig points out, sugar and high-fructose corn syrup are certainly not 'acute toxins' of the kind the FDA typically regulates and the effects of which can be studied over the course of days or months. The question is whether they're 'chronic toxins,' which means 'not toxic after one meal, but after 1,000 meals.'"[8] My premise is that sugar is toxic, but it can take those "1,000 meals" or years for some people to see the damage. For others like me, it can show up early on in life.

The scientists who believe that sugar is a uniquely toxic carbohydrate argue that its toxicity is connected with its metabolism in the liver. Consuming sugar too much or too long increases VLDL (unhealthy cholesterol) and triglycerides. The higher triglycerides cause a spike in apoB and LDL-P. ApoB is the primary protein of lipoproteins such as very low-density lipoprotein (VLDL) and low-density lipoprotein (LDL, the "bad cholesterol"), and it is involved in lipid (fat) metabolism. LDL-P is a measurement of the actual number of LDL particles, which is now considered a better predictor of cardiovascular risk than LDL-C. Insulin resistance is also worsened by sugar consumption.[9] Epidemiological studies and esteemed clinical evidence indict sugar when it comes to metabolic syndrome, type 2 diabetes, and cardiovascular disease.[10]

HER AHA MOMENT REGARDING SUGAR

Tonight, I got stupid and ate a portion of a gluten-free, sugar-laden cupcake. Thirty minutes later, my heart is pounding, twice as fast as usual. I was skipping heartbeats (not unusual for me). I've done this all my life, but amazingly though, not since the cleanse (The Juice Lady's 30-Day Detox Challenge). Sugar sure is poison.

—Agalia

To the Scorecard: Sugar Toxicity Unraveled

Americans eat most of their sugar in the form of refined white sugar, evaporated cane sugar, and high-fructose corn syrup. So what is a molecule of sugar anyway? Should you care to know, it's a bond between a glucose molecule and a fructose molecule—two simple sugars with the same chemistry. That's what people ate until the 1960s. Then along came the corn industry alternative, which produced a cheap conversion of corn-derived glucose into fructose. That heralded the birth of the high-fructose corn syrup (HFCS) industry. HFCS is made up of fructose (55 percent), glucose (42 percent), and other sugars (3 percent). Since fructose is nearly twice as sweet as glucose, you don't need as much to make a product sweet. Out of the cornfield, an inexpensive syrup and a cheap alternative to sucrose was born. They dumped it into nearly everything they could.

Your cells have a goal: to convert fructose and glucose into energy. They prefer fructose and glucose over sucrose, which is a rather bulky molecule. Your intestinal enzymes have to work harder on sucrose to split it into fructose and glucose. The end game is that all of your cells convert glucose into energy except your liver cells. They convert fructose to energy. That means fructose conversion depends on one very hardworking organ with a lot of other responsibilities, so fructose puts a lot of stress and strain on the liver.

When we eat ample amounts of fructose, the liver can start crying for help. With so much energy expended on fructose conversion, not much is left for other functions. On top of that fructose metabolism creates a boatload of toxins and waste products such as uric acid. And guess what! This shoots up blood pressure and causes ailments such as gout. (Rarely does anyone ever tell a gout sufferer that fructose could be the root cause.) It's also linked to kidney stones.

People often ask me if oxalate-rich dark leafy greens such as spinach can cause kidney stones. I have not found research supporting that premise. But there is plenty of evidence that sugar, especially fructose, can set people up for kidney stones.

One South African study reports that soda pop "exacerbates urine conditions that can lead to calcium oxalate kidney stone problems."[11] And here's another point to consider: sugar can "increase kidney size and produce pathological changes in your kidneys, such as the formation of kidney stones."[12]

Another consequence of eating too much fructose is fatty liver. Well, it's not just fructose; it's any sugar. But fructose has been shown to produce fat in your liver faster than any other type of sugar. By a process known as lipogenesis, fructose and other sugars create fat in the liver. If you eat enough fructose, little fat droplets start collecting in your liver cells. Suddenly, you get a disturbing diagnosis—nonalcoholic fatty liver disease! And you say, "what?" This is happening to younger and younger people. With this condition, the liver appears like the liver of someone who drinks excessive amounts of alcohol.[13] Research has also linked fatty liver to insulin resistance—a condition where cells become less responsive to insulin than normal cells. This puts strain on the pancreas and causes it to lose the ability to regulate blood glucose levels.[14]

"Virtually unknown before 1980, nonalcoholic fatty liver disease now affects up to 30% of adults in the United States and other developed countries, and between 70% and 90% of those who are obese or who have diabetes."[15] If you catch it early on and stop eating fructose and other forms of sugar, along with eating a diet that supports liver health, it is reversible. If you continue with your sugar-rich diet, "at some point...the liver can become inflamed. This can cause low-grade damage known as nonalcoholic steatohepatitis (*steato* meaning fat and *hepatitis* meaning liver inflammation). If the inflammation becomes severe, it can lead to cirrhosis—an accumulation of scar tissue and...degeneration of liver function."[16]

Sugar makes us fat. That's not new news. But did you know that it promotes visceral fat—a type of fat that forms around organs and in the abdominal region? This fat has a direct connection with heart disease.[17] *The New England Journal of Medicine* (2010) published an article showing that people with nonalcoholic fatty liver disease are more likely to have a buildup of cholesterol-filled plaque in their arteries, to develop cardiovascular disease, and to die from it.[18]

High-Fructose Corn Syrup: It's NOT Just Corn

Do you remember those TV commercials that began around 2008 to educate the public that HFCS is natural and safe? They featured a healthy-looking young woman in a cornfield saying, "But it's just corn." HFCS is anything but "just corn."

I found a post online in my search for information about HFCS that represents probably millions of people who have suffered the effects of this very toxic form of sugar. This is Victor's sad story of what high-fructose corn syrup and sugar did to his mother.

> My mother died from pancreatic cancer on October 18, 2009. She arrived in the United States from Ukraine in 1977, a healthy, slim thirty-five-year-old woman. No one in our family history had diabetes, or cancer. She had never had a soft drink before (really). She thought it was gross at first, but then got used to it. Yet after being exposed to GMO foods, corn syrup, cornstarch, and HFCS...for ten years, she developed diabetes, gained a lot of weight, began suffering from severe mental disorders...then ultimately [died] of pancreatic [cancer].[19]
>
> —VICTOR

The claim that corn syrup is fine if consumed in moderation is very appealing to many people. We all want to think we can have a little bit of nearly anything and be OK. But how closely can we walk the line before falling into the sticky abyss? Here's the truth: corn syrup has snuck into many foods we eat on a regular basis, such as cereals, sauces, peanut butter, yogurt, salad dressing, crackers, cookies, processed meats, energy bars...you name it. Unless we read labels all the time—and that means shopping with a magnifying glass so we can read the small print—we will never know it's there.

HFCS is cheap and has a long shelf life, making it very attractive to food manufacturers but not so attractive to the consumer. Unlike refined sugar, it contributes to overeating because it interferes with the brain's communication with leptin, the hormone that tells your brain that your stomach is full. It "may even trigger continued hunger pangs."[20] But there is something even more disturbing to consider: when HFCS is heated to just 120 degrees (that's very low), it can form a toxic chemical called hydroxymethylfurfural (HMF), which can kill honeybees. Studies in Sweden have "linked HMF to DNA damage in humans."[21] But that's not all. When we eat HFCS, it breaks down to next-generation metabolites—substances that are potentially more harmful than the original HFCS.

Researchers at Rutgers University discovered reactive carbonyls in beverages made with HFCS, which are free radicals linked to tissue damage, the onset of diabetes, and diabetes complications. Researcher Chi-Tang Ho estimates that "a single can of soda contains about five times the concentration of reactive carbonyls than the concentration found in the blood of an adult person with diabetes."[22]

Harvard School of Public Health says the breakdown of fructose in the liver can contribute to the following:

- Elevated triglycerides
- Increased harmful LDL (bad cholesterol)
- The buildup of fat around organs (visceral fat)
- Increased blood pressure
- Insulin-resistance, a precursor to diabetes
- Increased production of free radicals, energetic compounds that can damage DNA and cells.[23]

Other Types of Sugar That Don't Fight Fair

Though many people in the health field have singled out fructose as the black sheep of the sugar family, other forms of sugar are also questionable. Even if fructose is the foremost sugar to be blamed for obesity and diabetes, we must eat less sugar in all forms. Why? Sweets and sugar-enhanced foods are responsible for people eating far more food than they need. It might be a bit hard to swallow, but many of our favorite flavored coffee drinks, ice cream, yogurt, special desserts, energy bars, snacks, muffins, cereals, and energy drinks overwhelm the body with more sugar than it can metabolize. Many premade smoothies, frozen yogurt, and fruit juices all contain large amounts of sugar that will be readily absorbed into our system. To take in sugar in these liquid forms is like mainlining this stuff.

For over four hundred years sugar was a European luxury. That all changed when manufacturing made this white delicacy afford-able for the masses. We have Christopher Columbus to thank (or blame) for bringing sugarcane to the New World in 1493. Europeans established sugarcane plantations in the sixteenth and seventeenth centuries in the West Indies and South America. Not surprisingly, between the eighteenth and nineteenth centuries in England, sugar consumption increased by 1,500 percent. By the mid-nineteenth century Americans and Europeans considered refined sugar a necessity.

Today sugar in one of its many forms is added to almost all pro-cessed foods. We've even become generous about using it to sweeten many so-called healthy and whole foods. We call it "organic cane sugar" in the health food market. It's still sugar.

Many of us are "sugar babies"—we've been raised on this sweet stuff. Sweeteners are (and have been for a long time) in everything—from medicines to our morning cereal. Drinking soda is like drinking liquid candy. You'll find sugar, often in the form of HFCS, in fruit juices, sports drinks, and most processed foods such as lunch meats, cheese spreads, and crackers. Sugar is even in some of the most popular energy bars and thin bars. And now most infant formula has sugar; two popular brands tested had 13.5 and 12.4 grams per serving.[24] We're a nation choking on a gummy bear!

Today for an average American, more calories come from sugar than any other single food. What a difference a century or two makes! In the 1700s an average person ate about four pounds of sugar each year. By 1800 the average amount of sugar people ate was about eighteen pounds per person per year. In 1900 consumption had risen to ninety pounds of sugar a year for each person. But in the last century sugar consumption doubled again. In 2009 more than 50 percent of Americans ate one-half pound of sugar each day, which translates to about 180 pounds of sugar each year![25]

The Sweetest Poison of Them All

Refined sugar depletes your body of important vitamins and minerals because of the demands it makes on your entire system in digestion, detoxification, and elimination.

> In 1957, Dr. William Coda Martin tried to answer the question: When is a food a food and when is it a poison? His working definition of "poison" was: "Medically: Any substance applied to the body, ingested or developed within the body, which causes or may cause disease. Physically: Any substance which inhibits the activity of a catalyst which is a minor substance, chemical or enzyme that activates a reaction." The dictionary gives an even broader definition for "poison": "to exert a harmful influence on, or to pervert."

> Dr. Martin classified refined sugar as a poison because it
> has been depleted of its life forces, vitamins and minerals.[26]

Eating sugar every day produces an overacidic condition in your body. This means that minerals are leeched from various parts of the body to remedy the imbalance. For example, calcium is often pulled from the bones and teeth to protect the delicate pH of the blood. That means bones weaken; teeth may crack or decay. Sugar also causes fat to be deposited in organs, such as the heart, liver, and kidneys. Then the organs slow down and weaken. As more fat is produced, more of it accumulates in and around the organs. Blood pressure may go up. The circulatory and lymphatic systems become distressed. The immune system is compromised and unable to deal with harmful invaders or adverse situations, whether it's extreme cold, heat, viruses, bacteria, or microbes.

Could You Have Sugar Brain?

Sugar affects the brain. How often have you forgotten the name of the movie star from a movie you liked? Maybe the name of the restaurant where you had a fabulous meal on a vacation? Or what is the brand name of those comfy boots you got last year? Could it be sugar that is to blame? Glutamic acid, a compound found in many vegetables, is your key to a finely tuned, well-functioning brain. B vitamins play a key role in breaking down glutamic acid into complementary compounds that produce good brain responses. B vitamins are manufactured by friendly bacteria in the intestinal tract. When you eat refined sugar, the opportunistic bacteria like Candida albicans proliferate and outnumber the good bacteria; they weaken and die. This allows the opportunistic bacteria to thrive. Then our supply of B vitamins diminishes. And so the circle goes as our health spirals down.

Sugar can make us sleepy and lethargic during the day (and keep us awake at night). We may lose our ability to calculate, and our memory gets foggy. In all, it's worse than a flat-tire day. A 2012 study on rats, conducted by researchers at UCLA, found that a diet high in fructose "...hinders learning and memory by literally slowing down the brain. The researchers found that rats who over-consumed fructose had damaged synaptic activity in the brain, meaning that communication among brain cells was impaired."[27]

High-sugar and high-carb foods can also mess up the brain neurotransmitters that are responsible for mood stability. And why do we eat this stuff anyway? Our bodies seem to desire it, even in our brains: sugar stimulates the release of the "mood-boosting neurotransmitter serotonin."[28] This might sound like a good thing, but according to Dr. Datis Kharrazian, "constantly over-activating these serotonin pathways can deplete our limited supplies of this neurotransmitter, which can contribute to symptoms of depression."[29]

In particular, teenagers are affected by sugar and what it does in the body. A recent study using adolescent mice, conducted at Emory University School of Medicine, found that sugar-filled diets demonstrated a common link with depression and anxiety.[30] However, older people, even seniors, are also vulnerable. A 2013 study found that insulin resistance and higher blood glucose levels—two indicators of diabetes—are linked with a greater risk of neurodegenerative disorders like Alzheimer's.[31]

You can read much more about sugar brain in chapter 4.

Toxic Sweet Soup

I'm part Norwegian. I remember many holidays when "sweet soup" was served. It had a lot of dried fruit and sugar. Though that menu item has its own list of issues, that's not the sweet soup I'm talking about here. The internal environment of the body's "soup" includes tissue fluid, which bathes all our cells, along with blood and lymph. The composition of this interstitial fluid must remain constant if cells are to stay alive and healthy. Sugar and sweetened foods are very acidic, and colas and other soft drinks are highly acidic.

When your blood becomes acidic, the body deposits acidic substances (toxins) into your cells to make sure the blood remains at proper pH balance. Acids can collect in tissue fluids, causing the cells to become acidic and toxic. This decreases oxygen levels at the cellular level. This is damaging for DNA and respiratory enzymes. The tissue fluids can become a murky soup of toxins and wastes. The cells begin to "choke" on this stuff. Some die. Other cells can become abnormal, or malignant.

Alkaline fluids hold oxygen; acidic fluids only carry small amounts of oxygen. If our fluids are too acidic, toxins won't be released from our cells into the blood, and the cells won't detoxify properly.

The lymphatic system, which is the body's waste elimination channel, is also affected. When it gets congested with waste, nothing moves well. When the lymph ceases to function properly and the collecting terminals (lymph nodes) become blocked, it's like a jam-up on the freeway. Lymph begins to back up into the system, creating a toxic, oxygen-deprived environment that promotes cancer and other degenerative diseases and disorders.

Toxic lymph can build up for a long time in the system, where it becomes thicker, gel-like, stagnant, and overloaded with toxic waste. When the lymph fluid becomes sluggish, it changes in appearance from a water-like consistency to milk-like, becoming a breeding ground for disease.

Sugar Wrap

Sugar is not responsible for all this toxicity or all physical ailments; there are many contributing factors to toxic interstitial fluids, blood, lymph, cells, and a variety of physical ailments. But in America sugar is a major contributing factor. And when you try to get off the sweets, you find out just how addictive they are. But you may say, "How much harm can one little candy bar, one can of soda, or a cookie do? Okay, empty calories, cavities in the teeth, fattening… I know all about that." But today's research argues that sugar isn't just a high-caloric substitute for nourishing foods; it's a toxin in and of itself. It can wreak havoc on your health, making you sick, over-weight, tired, and depressed. And it's addictive. We'll learn just how addictive it is in the next chapter.

Chapter 2

SWEET TOOTH OR ADDICTION?

H OW MANY TIMES have you had the urge—the unstoppable craving—to get something sweet, right now? How often have you experienced yearning for a cookie that's so strong you eat half the dough before you get those little guys baked, or desire for ice cream that will get you into your car at night on a mission for your favorite flavor? What about the urge for a soda that will motivate you to walk up and down fifty steps at an arena for your favorite bubbly drink? Are we weak-willed or are we hard-wired to want sweet things?

Sweet Deception: The Lure of the Ice Cream Cone

Researchers in one study concluded that cravings for ice cream were similar to a drug addicts' cravings for their drug of choice. They found that when participants ate ice cream, the brain wanted more, just like that of a regular cocaine user. Their study, which was published online in the *American Journal of Clinical Nutrition*, added weight to other studies showing that people can become addicted to sweets.

Dr. Kyle Burger, with the Oregon Research Institute, noted, "Overeating 'high-fat' or 'high-sugar' foods appeared to change how the brain responded and in turn downgraded the mental reward."[1]

He went on to say that this "down-regulation pattern is seen with frequent drug use, where the more an individual uses the drug, the less reward they receive from using it."[2]

The American Society of Addiction Medicine says that "addiction is a primary, chronic disease of brain reward, motivation, memory, and related circuitry. Dysfunction in these circuits leads to characteristic biological, psychological, social, and spiritual manifestations. This is reflected in an individual pathologically pursuing reward and/or relief by substance use [and abuse] and other behaviors."[3]

What does all that research mean for you? Your pleasure center can get triggered by sugar just like that of a drug addict and... voila!—you have a full-blown sugar addiction. Why should you care about being addicted? You would probably like to lose a few pounds, right? You may also want to improve your health. Sugar is your opponent on both fronts.

Addiction, the Brain, and Pleasure Seeking

What is addiction anyway? In simple terms, sugar addiction is the compulsory eating of sugar. The experts say, "Addiction is characterized by inability to consistently abstain, impairment in behavioral control, craving, diminished recognition of significant problems with one's behaviors and interpersonal relationships, and a dysfunctional emotional response. Like other chronic diseases, addiction often involves cycles of relapse and remission. Without treatment or engagement in recovery activities"—and a turning from your old ways—"addiction is progressive and can result in disability or premature death."[4]

Here's what's going on in your brain. Sugar induces reactions in the nucleus accumbens (a region in the basal forebrain). Regular consumption of sugar can result in addiction because sugar targets this area of the brain. Like drugs, sugar can cause the neurons in the brain to release dopamine—the feel-good chemical. This makes people crave more of the "drug" to regain that pleasurable sensation. Sugar activates this reward pathway. Evidence indicates that sugary foods create stronger cravings than other types of food, causing people to want more and more sweets. Why? The orbito-frontal cortex, the area in the front of our brains where we process rewards, is activated when we eat sugar.[5] We get addicted to that reward response, so in other words, we're hooked on pleasure-seeking through food.

After eating sugar, the pancreas secretes insulin to distribute it in the blood to the cells. Subsequently, blood sugar drops, energy depletes, and some people experience a shaky feeling, which makes them want more sugar to feel "normal" again. This has been likened to the withdrawal-and-craving cycle typical of drug abuse. Sugar addiction is considered by some health professionals to be the most widespread addiction on the planet.

Why people get addicted to sugar is as varied as the stars. The negative feeling or symptom that an addiction temporarily relieves can be just about anything—anger, rage, fear, terror, anxiety, or grief. It could be boredom, apathy, loneliness, depression, or frustration. Sugar offers us a little momentary high—enough to relieve feelings of being out of sorts. This can lead to an addictive lifestyle.

Your sugar addiction may connect with a trauma, loss, or even a pleasant memory in the past. Perhaps your mother or father gave you sweets to cheer you up when you were teased at school, or your dentist gave you candy as a reward for being a good patient. It's a setup for sure. Now, as an adult, each time that you eat something sweet, you recall the good feelings. This becomes an emotional trigger that worsens sugar addiction.

It is believed that for some people, eating sweets is an attempt to bring sweetness into their lives. I believe that was true for me. As I mentioned in the introduction, my mother died when I was six years old. I was overwhelmingly addicted to sweets as a child. I would eat the whole thing, whatever it was—a carton of ice cream, a batch of cookies, a bag of candy—and not quit until it was gone. I remember eating sweets until I was almost in a trance. I would have mainlined the stuff if I could. Once I would start eating something sweet, it was very difficult for me to stop. I haven't eaten sugar in decades, but I still remember the feelings of satisfaction and desire for more and more sugar.

Rats Hooked on Oreo Cookies!

Studies on sugar being as addictive as cocaine or heroin have placed sugar at the forefront of a hot debate. A study published in the *American Journal of Clinical Nutrition* indicates that sugar and high-glycemic foods can be very addictive.[6] David Ludwig, author of *Ending the Food Fight*, along with his colleagues at Harvard, showed that foods with higher sugar content can trigger that special region in the brain—the "ground zero" for addictions like gambling, drug abuse, or sexual addiction.[7]

In 2013 Connecticut College released the Oreo cookie study. An article summarizing the research was titled "Research Shows Oreos Are Just as Addictive as Drugs," but it could just as truth-fully been titled: "Drugs Are No More Addictive Than Oreos." The specific drugs included in the study were cocaine and morphine (heroin is an opiate drug that is synthesized from morphine).[8] James DiNicolantonio, a cardiovascular research scientist at St. Luke's Mid-America Heart Institute in Kansas City, Missouri, said that "even when you get the rats hooked on IV cocaine, once you introduce sugar, almost all of them switch to the sugar."[9]

Another 2013 study titled "Sugar Addiction: Pushing the Drug-Sugar Analogy to the Limit" gives evidence that sweeteners can "induce reward and cravings that are comparable in magnitude to those induced by addictive drugs."[10] In other words, rewarding yourself with something sweet can be as powerful as addictive drugs like cocaine—and can be even more rewarding than those drugs! Sweet rewards—on a neurobiological level—appear to be more attractive than those of cocaine.[11] The research team of a 2007 study found that regardless of caloric content—sugar versus saccharin (Sweet'N Low), the intense pleasure of sweetness seems to be more "addictive than even the sensitization and intoxication brought about by cocaine, which mainstream society still recognizes as being much more harmful than sugar."[12]

It is apparent that in part sugar addition is the reason nearly 70 percent of Americans are overweight and half of the US population is either pre-diabetic or already has type 2 diabetes. It's not lack of willpower or a deficiency of personal responsibility—although these aspects may all play a part in overeating sweets for many people. Scientists have looked at the many and varied reasons the pleasure center can light up like a scoreboard such as taste, smell, or sight. When it does, we know our sugar attraction is alive and well.

Anatomy of Sugar Addiction

Several decades ago I read a book by William Dufty titled *Sugar Blues*. The author wrote about the addictive properties of sugar and the ways in which our nation's declining health can be blamed on our consumption of sweets.[13] As a society we essentially ignored this book and the warning to cut back on our sugar consumption.

But many of the ideas he set forth in this book, which came out years ago, have been confirmed by today's scientific discoveries. We now know that various neuroendocrine pathways are actually activated by sugar. The often-joked-about "sweet tooth" and our continual sugar cravings prove to us how these pathways can drive our obsessive addiction to sweets.

Here's what the experts have to say:

> "In most mammals, including rats and humans, sweet receptors evolved in ancestral environments poor in sugars and are thus not adapted to high concentrations of sweet tastants," wrote the author of another study involving bees, which experienced cocaine-withdrawal-type symptoms when their sweet floral supplies were taken away from them. 'The supranormal [beyond the range of the normal or scientifically explainable] stimulation of these receptors by sugar-rich diets, such as those now widely available in modern societies, would generate a supranormal reward signal in the brain, with the potential to override self-control mechanisms and thus to lead to addiction."[14]

DiNicolantonio says that a "consumption threshold" must be reached over a period of time to alter the brain's neurochemistry. Then when sugar is stopped, people experience "dopamine depletion and sugar withdrawal symptoms."

> "You get this intense release of dopamine upon acute ingestion of sugar. After you continuously consume it, those dopamine receptors start becoming down-regulated—there's less of them, and they're less responsive," he said. "That can lead to ADHD-like symptoms...but it can also lead to a mild state

of depression because we know that dopamine is that reward neurotransmitter."[15]

Dr. Mark Hyman commented on a randomized, blind, crossover study that proved the science of sugar addiction.

> They took 12 overweight or obese men between the ages of 18 and 35 and gave each a low-sugar or low glycemic–index (37 percent) milkshake, and then, four hours later, they measured the activity of the brain region (*nucleus accumbens*) that controls addiction. They also measured blood sugar and hunger.
>
> Then, days later, they had them drink another milkshake, but they switched the milkshakes. They were designed to taste and look exactly the same in every way except in how much and how quickly it spiked blood sugar. The second milk was designed to be high in sugar with a high glycemic index (84 percent). The shakes had the same number of calories, protein, fat, and carbohydrate....The participants didn't know which milkshake they were getting and their mouth couldn't tell the difference, but their brains could.
>
> Each participant received a brain scan and blood tests for glucose and insulin after each version of the milkshake. They were their own control group. Without exception, they all had the same response. The high sugar or glycemic index milkshake caused a spike in blood sugar and insulin and an increase in hunger and cravings four hours after the shake....
>
> ...When the high glycemic shake was consumed, the *nucleus accumbens* lit up like a Christmas tree. This pattern occurred in every single participant and was statistically significant.[16]

Another reason for sugar addiction is an overgrowth of yeast known as Candida albicans, which thrives on sugar. When people stop eating it, the yeasts start to die off. This triggers a craving for sweets, since the yeasts want more of their favorite food. Also many people are actually addicted to the alcohol the yeasts produce. The alcohol gives people a bit of a "high" all the time and slightly numbs consciousness, which reduces feelings of depression, anxiety, anger, and frustration. All this makes it hard to go on the "Candida Diet" and get the yeast under control.

Sugar—A Great Marketing Strategy

Who wants us to have our eating habits under control anyway? Certainly not the food manufacturers. They dump sugar in nearly everything knowing they'll get us addicted to their product. Historically, refined sugar entered the market about the same time as coffee, tea, distilled alcohol, and chocolate. Over time, they have all been manipulated to be stronger, more addictive, more toxic, and more injurious than the originals that were consumed centuries ago, or even just decades ago. With sugar, the effects are so subtle that very few are aware they are being affected by it. Sugar, like drugs, affects the mind, perception, and mood—how we think, move, and feel. Sugar consumption can cause us to feel euphoric and like we've had an upper followed by a downer. White sugar is similar to ecstasy, opiates, LSD, and methamphetamines, and it affects brain chemicals, creating a false sense of feeling that everything is OK even when it is not. The consumer gets withdrawal symptoms when it is not available.

Sugar, similarly to marijuana, opiates, tobacco, and meth, works on the same dopamine receptors in the brain. When dopamine becomes imbalanced, we can experience lack of interest, motivation, and willpower; loss of joy; depression; and listlessness. It can contribute to ADHD. It also promotes taurine and serotonin deficiencies. Therefore we are left craving more and more of the sweet substances that help us feel back on track again, at least for a few moments.[17]

Food manufacturers are smart. They know sugar is addictive, so they add it to fast food, snack foods, and almost anything in a package because it sells. A great deal of the advertising of sweet things is aimed at children. Ad campaigns also target young parents with captivating advertising for foods such as sugary cereal and sweet drinks. Early in life, many people get addicted to products containing sweeteners. Sugar is also in foods that don't even taste sweet, such as tomato sauce and deli meats. Sales soar and companies profit. But what toll does it take on our bodies? Science has shown, beyond any doubt, that sugar in all its myriad forms is creating a nation of addicts and sick people.

The Bliss Point

Dr. Joseph Mercola has reported that food production companies spend a great deal of money to learn the exact scientific calculations for combining ingredients in just the right way to make people crave their products. This is actually called the bliss point. Dr. Howard Moskowitz, a Harvard-trained mathematician whose nickname is Dr. Bliss due to his work in this field, designs and implements testing procedures of people's reactions in order to find just the right amount of sugar to make them crave a product on a regular basis. He calls it the "Goldilocks" zone, and his work has made the sugar industry literally billions of dollars.[18]

Dr. Bliss was originally hired by the U.S. Army to research how to get soldiers to eat more unappetizing army rations in the field. The troops weren't eating enough food because, according to the men, it was "so boring." They would toss the half-eaten rations away.

When Dr. Bliss discovered what he called "sensory-specific satiety," he learned that big flavors could overwhelm the brain and actually suppress the desire to stop eating. Satiety—the feeling of having had enough to eat—can be overridden by flavors that tell your brain to keep eating. Bliss then found the magic formula—just the right amount of sugar, salt, and fat that would bring the soldiers to the bliss point. In our modern times and armed with this knowledge, the processed food industry has now added sugar (and salt and fat) to nearly everything to get you to eat more of their products. This is what makes processed foods so addictive.[19]

PRODUCTS WITH A HIGH SUGAR CONTENT THAT ARE NOT OFTEN CONSIDERED HIGH IN SUGAR

- BBQ sauce—There are 13 grams of sugar in 2 tablespoons.
- Fruit yogurt—There are 19 grams of sugar in many single-serving containers. It tastes like dessert because it is dessert.
- Sweet and sour chicken—There are 19 grams of sugar in many servings.
- Spaghetti sauce—One-half cup may contain as much as 12 grams of sugar. (Plus the pasta turns rapidly to sugar because it's digested so quickly.)
- Sodas—One 8-ounce soda can offers 29 sugar grams; a 20-ounce soda can contain 65 grams of sugar. (Well, this one you probably are aware of—just wanted you to show how much sugar is actually there.)
- Dried fruit—One-third cup can have as much as 24 grams of sugar; many manufacturers add sugar.
- Gummy worms—There are 44 grams of sugar in every 10 worms.
- Energy bars—One bar can pack in 12 grams or more of sugar.
- Energy drinks—Some pack in as much as 83 grams of sugar.[20]

The food industry has hidden the truth about sugar for many years. Their primary goal is to find ways to hook you and make you more addicted to their products. They do not care in the least about the consequences to your health. In 2012 science journalist Gary Taubes partnered with Cristin Kearns Couzens to write "Big Sugar's Sweet Little Lies," an article for *Mother Jones* magazine. They wrote: "For 40 years, the sugar industry's priority has been to shed doubt on studies suggesting its product makes people sick. On federal panels, industry-funded scientists cited industry-funded studies to dismiss sugar as a culprit."[21] There is evidence from as far back as the 1970s that sugar has a role in heart disease. But then, if that news was widely broadcast, the sugar industry would have lost billions. So they blamed it all on fat.[22] We didn't have a fat lobby to fight that one, so the message stuck.

Sweeteners are also the biggest contributor to obesity, which has more than doubled in America since 1975. Eating too much sugar and refined carbs that easily turn to sugar has been implicated in insulin resistance, metabolic syndrome, and diabetes. Both type 1 and type 2 diabetics should completely avoid sugar in all forms as a way of stabilizing blood sugar and controlling the disease. Foods for diabetics is big business, even though many of the products are not good for diabetics at all because they contain some form of sugar, including artificial sweeteners.

Eating sugary food first causes spikes in blood sugar levels, and then causes dips, which can lead to sleepiness, tiredness, light-headedness, and in extreme cases, lack of coordination and slurred speech. Sugar is also a major contributing factor in hypoglycemia, insulin resistance, and metabolic syndrome. The only hope of controlling blood sugar imbalance is through a sugar-free diet, yet many diabetics and other people with sugar metabolism problems have become so addicted to sugar that they cannot give it up, even when they face the possibility of losing a toe, a foot, or even a leg. Dr. David Kessler, two-term head of the FDA, shows scientifically how our addiction to sugar might be the downfall of all Western civilization. You can listen to his interview at https://www.youtube.com/watch?v=QI2h4cBCpoA.

Sugar has a lot of calories, which has prompted many manufacturers of processed foods to develop low-calorie foods made with artificial sweeteners like aspartame (NutraSweet) and sucralose (Splenda). But artificial sweeteners are even worse for your health than sugar, and studies show they actually cause people to eat more sweets and gain more weight than those eating or drinking beverages made with sugar. As we saw earlier with one study, Sweet'N Low had the same effect on the pleasure center (addictive center) of the brain as did sugar.

A PASTOR'S ADDICTION TO DOUGHNUTS

Pastor William Joseph says he hated his father's alcoholism, but it turns out he wasn't that different. In his *Guideposts* story "Giving His Addiction Up to God," William writes, "I didn't need the doughnuts, but having a special treat helped. Nothing wrong with that. So why had I lied to the Krispy Kreme guy? That was what alcoholics and druggies did, right?...I didn't want anyone to notice how many doughnuts I ate."

William had worked up to where he would sometimes eat four dozen doughnuts at a time. He would probably have kept on this addictive path, he said, were it not for an infection in his blood due to untreated diabetes. His doctor told him had he not come in for treatment that day, he would have been in serious trouble, maybe even life-threatening.[23]

When he faced his addiction, he finally called his dad, who had been sober since he started AA. He asked his dad what he did to make the cravings go away. "You turn it over," he said. "You give it up to God. You pray and you fight for your sobriety every day. Honesty is the key."[24]

William says, "Both of us had been chasing something you can't put in a bottle or bake into a doughnut. We were trying to fill a hole in our lives, to satisfy a spiritual longing." William got honest with his wife and children about his addiction. "It wasn't easy," he said, "but prayer and honesty, love and understanding saw me through. I haven't touched a doughnut in over twenty years."[25]

Ten Signs You Might Be Addicted to Sugar

1. You have belly fat.

2. You can't stop eating sweets once you start.

3. You crave sugar and carbs.

4. You rely on sweets for emotional support or comfort.

5. You have high blood sugar.

6. You eat sweets even if you're not hungry.

7. You get excited about desserts, sweet drinks, or sugary snacks.

8. You feel embarrassed about eating all the sweets you consume, or you hide them.

9. You feel agitated or irritable, can't sleep well, or suffer withdrawal symptoms if you don't get sweets, refined carbohydrates, or starch each day.

10. You feel out of control when it comes to your sweet tooth.

Take the Sugar Addiction Quiz

You may like your sweets, but are you really addicted to sugar? Take the quiz and learn the truth.

1. Do you want to eat something sweet when you've had a bad day?

   Yes

   No

2. Do you eat something sweet every day such as cookies, pastries, chocolate, pie, ice cream, or candy?

   Yes

   No

3. Do you experience a sense of happiness, excitement, or relief when you eat sweets?

   Yes

   No

4. Do you feel good while you are indulging in sweets but worse afterward?

   Yes

   No

5. Do sweets have control over you?

   Yes

   No

6. Do you ever travel far, go out late at night, or stay up late to make sweets, or do you ever overcome obstacles to make or purchase sweets?

Yes

No

7. When you see pictures of desserts, does it stir up emotions or desires in you?

Yes

No

8. Do you feel guilty or remorseful after eating sweets?

Yes

No

9. Do you have a hard time resisting dessert at parties, get-togethers, or restaurants?

Yes

No

10. Do you typically eat sweets when you are alone?

Yes

No

11. Do you eat sweets to the point of feeling sick?

Yes

No

12. Do you find yourself thinking about sweets during the day or planning what sweet treat you will have next?

Yes

No

13. When you eat sweets, does this cause you to want more?

Yes

No

14. Do you stockpile sweet snacks or desserts?

Yes

No

15. Do you have a hard time stopping at just one cookie or one piece of pie?

Yes

No

16. Do you ever try and fail to stop eating sweets or drastically reduce the amount of sweets you eat?

Yes

No

17. When you eat sweets, do you feel out of control?

Yes

No

18. Do you experience withdrawal symptoms when you go without sweets for a while?

Yes

No

19. Do you lie or try to hide the amount of sweets you eat?

Yes

No

20. Does it feel like it's never enough? For instance, do you eat something sweet once and then want it over and over again?

Yes

No

21. Are you concerned that eating sugar will damage your health but you keep eating it anyway?

Yes

No

22. If you are alone with your favorite box, sack, or carton of sweets, would you eat the whole thing?

Yes

No

23. Do you often tell yourself this is the "last time I am doing this," and then overeat sweets because you thought it would be the last time?

Yes

No

24. Do you feel like it isn't a celebration unless you have something sweet?

Yes

No

25. Do you ever sacrifice health foods for something sweet?

Yes

No

26. Would your friends describe you as having a sweet tooth?

Yes

No

Interpretation of the Quiz

If you answered yes to four or more of these questions, then you most likely have an addiction to sweets. It's time to stop deceiving yourself, if you have been, and get help.

If you answered yes to between one and three of these questions, then you may develop an addiction later.

Zero yes answers means you don't have a problem.

The Eyes Have It!

A radio host I listened to while I was writing this chapter said she had just seen a picture of a smoothie and now she was craving one. Restaurants know the power of seeing desserts. There's a reason they come to your table with a scrumptious tray of sweets. You may have said ten times that evening that you weren't going to have dessert, but it all skips out the door when your sight beholds the chef's lovely creations. So what's going on? Your eyes have connected with the pleasure center of your brain and overpowered your resolve.

Advertisers know that sugar addictions are triggered by environmental cues. Watching a TV commercial with a child licking an ice cream cone, viewing cinnamon rolls popping out of the oven, or seeing someone eating chocolates can cause you to want to start eating it yourself. Over time it will become a habit to simply reach for sugary foods with visual cues. It's similar to what happens with addictive drugs. A classic example is a motivated person who goes through drug rehab like a champ, but then she returns to her former environment and friends, and suddenly she finds herself craving drugs again. What happened? Environmental cues.[26]

Numerous studies have shown how the pleasure center of the brain lights up in response to images of sugary foods. Many studies use different foods for comparison, such as cheesecake or boiled vegetables, and they all show the same thing—sight creates the urge to eat sweets when it connects with the brain's pleasure center.

A Very Real Addiction

Only recently has sugar been thought of as a substance to which people can become addicted. While the studies with rats and people point to the neurochemical and biological effects of sugar, many health professionals remain skeptical about any clear connection between the body and sugar addiction. But those caught in its clutches know the truth—sugar can destroy one's life. It can affect us on every level, including spiritually. Are addiction and gluttony in the same category? Dante depicted gluttony in the third circle of the inferno. He showed people in this part of hell as punished by being held hostage in a putrid bog and forced to wallow in freezing rain and stinking sewage, with some forced to swallow it, representing the waste and corruption they had inflicted upon their own bodies. The vile sludge symbolized the personal degradation of a person who overindulges in food, drink, and other worldly pleasures and the glutton's selfishness and coldness.

Sugar dependence has three stages—bingeing, withdrawal, and craving. Sugar can cause the brain chemicals serotonin and dopamine to increase. These neurotransmitters are involved with pleasure, reward, and pain tolerance, so this makes sugar powerfully attractive. And because sugar is irresistible for many people, it is challenging to stop. Detoxing from sugar is what this book is about. I've developed a plan to help you get off sugar and cleanse your body (see chapter 9). Next, however, I'll look at how sugar impacts our health and well-being.

Chapter 3

THE MAIN EVENT: YOU VERSUS SUGAR

Y OU MAY BE in for a surprise. There are so many ways in which sugar affects us that it's almost staggering. It's time to get smart about this stuff. In this chapter I'll show you many of the ways it impacts your body. I'm actually amazed that this most poisonous substance has not made headline news. But I'm also aware that we have a powerful sugar lobby, so in that respect I'm not amazed. We're a nation gone wild on a sugar binge. Everyone should be warned of sugar's deleterious effects on the body, yet little warning is ever given.

If you go to a doctor regarding an illness, are you ever asked if you're eating sugar? Probably not. Your doctor may love sweets too. We dream about the chocolate or sweet-flavored latte we'll have on our break. We look forward to birthday cake or holiday pie. We drive out of our way to get our favorite ice cream or cupcake. Sweets are America's darling…but it's anything but sweet when it comes to our bodies and our health. Extra pudge is only the beginning. Disease all dressed up in white is what's lurking in the bottom of that sugar bowl.

In September 2013 Credit Suisse's Research Institute sounded the alarm regarding the overwhelming consequences of sugar on our health. This research group found that approximately "30%–40% of healthcare expenditures in the USA go to help address issues that are closely tied to the excess consumption of sugar."[1] Their calculations show that our nationwide sugar addiction is responsible for $1 trillion in annual health-care costs. That's a high price to pay for our Milk Duds, sweet cereals, sodas, coffee mochas, and cupcakes.

In the pages that follow, you'll see the many ways that sugar can adversely impact your health. This is not an exhaustive list by any means. Many doctors and health professionals believe that sugar in its many forms has been the demise of our nation's health.

Eleven Good Reasons to Hit Sugar Below the Belt

1. Sugar is a major contributor to inflammation.

Inflammation is a top cause of heart disease and nearly all other diseases. You can read more about inflammation in my book *The Juice Lady's Anti-Inflammation Diet.* Research has revealed disturbing links between sugar and inflammatory conditions. Inflammation has been identified as a major factor in most diseases, from cancer and diabetes to atherosclerosis and Alzheimer's.

Sugar plays a significant role in inflammation. It is believed sugar is a contributor to injuries deep inside the body, such as the blood vessels, where you don't see or feel it, yet this hidden form of inflammation can cause heart disease. Health professionals have only just begun to understand how sugar fans the flames of inflammation.

When it comes to heart disease, Walter Willett, MD, professor of epidemiology and nutrition at the Harvard School of Public Health (HSPH), says the type of *carbohydrates* you eat may be as important as the type of *fat*.[2] The more refined carbohydrates you eat, the more likely you are to be overloading your body with sugar. This causes you to slide down the inflammation highway.

Willett and his research team studied the diets and health

histories of more than 75,500 women who took part in the Nurses' Health Study. It was discovered that those who ate the highest amount of refined carbohydrates doubled their risk of a heart attack because sugar converts to triglycerides, and high triglycerides are a key indicator of heart disease.[3]

Did you know that high sugar diets stress the heart? It's true. When your blood sugar is high, your body produces more free radicals. These toxic molecules go on an excursion in your body, damaging cells and overstimulating your immune system responses. Left unchecked, this can inflame the lining of your blood vessels that lead to the heart.[4] Free radicals can inflame the brain, thyroid gland, pancreas, and just about any place in your body. Too much sugar can alert the body to send out extra immune system messengers—the cytokines, which are small cell proteins involved in cell signaling. The pro-inflammatory cytokines can fuel inflammation.

The less sugar you eat, the less inflammation you will experience, and the stronger your immune system will be to defend you against infectious and degenerative diseases.

2. Sugar will raise your cholesterol.

Do you want to reduce your risk of coronary heart disease? Reduce the amount of sugar in your diet. For years we were told it was fat that raised our cholesterol, but sugar is far worse. Research links sugar with unhealthy cholesterol and triglyceride levels.

The cholesterol that causes atherosclerosis, or plaque in your arteries, is mainly manufactured by your body, rather than the dietary cholesterol present in the foods you eat, explains cardiologist and cholesterol expert Dr. Seth Baum, founder of Preventive Cardiology.[5] "Even more confusing is that the amount of 'bad' cholesterol (known as LDL) in your blood is not as important as the number of LDL particles you create. LDL particles transport LDL cholesterol throughout your body. The more LDL particles in your blood, the more likely LDL cholesterol will penetrate your arteries, create plaque, and then cause the arterial problems, including inflammation, that can lead to heart attack and stroke."[6]

What increases LDL particles? Sugar.

In 2010 the *Journal of the American Medical Association* published a study based on data collected from 6,113 adults monitored over the course of ten years. The results of the study showed that people who ate the most sugar had the lowest HDL (good cholesterol) and the highest blood triglyceride levels. They reported that "people who ate the least sugar had the highest HDL and the lowest triglyceride levels. Eating large amounts of added sugar more than tripled the risk of having low HDL, which is a major risk factor for heart disease."[7]

Dr. Mark Hyman's article titled "Eggs Don't Cause Heart Attacks—Sugar Does" says, "Government eating guidelines have been wrong. We've been told to swap eggs for Cheerios. But that recommendation is dead wrong. In fact, it's very likely that this bad advice has killed millions of Americans."[8] A study published in *JAMA Internal Medicine*, with more than forty thousand participants, indicated that people who ate the most sugar had a fourfold increase in heart attack risk compared to those who ate the least amount of sugar.[9] Dr. Hyman cites the worst offenders as sugar-sweetened beverages such as sodas, fruit juices, sports drinks, sweetened teas, and coffees.[10]

Decades of research on sugar shows us that it's responsible for insulin resistance, high triglycerides, lower HDL, and elevated LDL, and it triggers inflammation, which is at the root of heart disease.[11] As a whole, the medical community keeps blaming saturated fat and cholesterol for heart disease. It's as ludicrous as drinking poison and expecting someone else to die. The hard facts point to sugar calories as being the worst calories we can eat. A 2013 study of more than 175 countries discovered that the risk of type 2 diabetes was not increased by consuming more *overall* calories. However, the risk was dramatically increased by eating more *sugar* calories.[12]

3. ADHD, hyperactivity, and autism are affected by sugar.

Perhaps the biggest reason to ditch sugar is the children. Sugar affects their mood and behavior in very adverse ways—irritability, hyperactivity, angry outbursts, and just plain bad mood. Every parent knows that allowing a child sugar or anything with ample amounts of sugar can dramatically change their behavior! But interestingly the medical community appears to be silent on this issue. Still there is no question that what your children eat and drink dramatically affects how they think, feel, and behave. One study done at the University of South Carolina discovered that the more sugar that hyperactive children ate, the more restless and destructive they grew.[13] A different study carried out at Yale University learned that high-sugar diets can create even worse attention in some ADHD children.[14]

About 10 percent of children are diagnosed with ADHD, and 2.7 million children are taking medications for this disorder. We need to start asking whether or not we are medicating a large number of children when we should actually be changing their diet. Sugar is toxic, and it will cause a toxic reaction in the brains of many children. A child's reaction can vary from acting hyper and demonstrating lack of focus to being argumentative.

"Sugar is poison because of the way the body metabolizes it. The sugar interferes with the respiration of the cells. They cannot get sufficient oxygen to survive and function normally.

In time, some of the cells die. This interferes with the function of a part of the body and is the beginning of degenerative disease." Excess sugar will interfere in the child's cognitive function and in his or her behavior in the classroom, at home, and with peers.[15]

Researchers who worked with mice bred to display autism-like behaviors found they could ease the behaviors with a low-sugar diet beginning with the animals' mothers during pregnancy.[16]

Sugar changes our behavior, our ability to pay attention, and how we learn. Studies about how sugar affects the behavior of children are contradictory, but it is generally accepted that some children and adults are far more sensitive to sugar than others. Their level of sugar sensitivity is in direct proportion to how they display behavioral issues, difficulties with maintaining focus and attention, and deterioration of learning ability. Based on the research, it seems that children may be more sensitive to sugar than adults. One study that compared how children and adults respond to sugar showed that the "adrenaline levels in children remained ten times higher than normal for up to five hours after a test dose of sugar."[17] Excess sugar also contributes to high adrenaline levels and low blood sugar levels, which produce abnormal behavior.

4. Sugar destroys your teeth.

This certainly isn't new news. Since we were kids we've all been told that sugar causes cavities. We know that sugar increases the bacteria in your mouth, which erodes enamel. Tooth erosion occurs when acid attacks tooth enamel. Once your saliva is acidic, it dissolves calcium from your tooth enamel in a process called demineralization. As this process continues, you'll lose enough tooth structure to develop a hole in your tooth. Some of the worst sugar offenders are mints, cough drops, and hard candies that you suck on. They have a unique demineralization effect because usually the candy or lozenge ends up sitting in one area of your mouth for a longer period of time and you get a concentrated buildup of acid on the teeth in that spot. Sticky candies like caramels are bad news too, because they stick to your teeth and saliva can't get to that part of your tooth to neutralize the acid or re-mineralize those teeth, causing a greater loss of calcium. Sports drinks and sodas can stick to your teeth for longer periods of time as well.[18] Also, avoid sugar-sweetened toothpaste.

5. Sugar causes aging and wrinkles.

For the last four decades, Americans have avoided fats and gorged on sugar. Sugar in the amount that the typical American eats continually upsets our body chemistry and causes the inflammatory process that leads to aging. Many times we don't even know we're eating sugar. It's hidden in packaging in many different forms: high-fructose corn syrup, corn syrup solids, sucrose, maltose, dextrose, fructose, glucose, galactose, and on it goes.

The less sugar you eat, the less inflammation and aging you'll have. Here's why: excessive sugar is a major cause of glycation—a process in which sugar binds to protein or fat and forms advanced glycation end products (AGEs). AGEs are inflammatory and are connected with type 2 diabetes, aging, and many diseases. Sugar is one of the major factors that increase production of AGEs inside your body. Along with oxidation, AGEs are a major contributor to looking older and getting sicker. Over time high blood sugar levels dramatically increase age-accelerated AGEs. This is why type 2 diabetics may often look older than their real age. But this age-accelerating effect is not just limited to diabetics.

Limiting or omitting sugar is a key to longevity. According to Dr.

Mercola, sugar molecules are the most damaging molecules to the body. He says:

> Fructose in particular is an extremely potent pro-inflammatory agent that creates AGEs and speeds up the aging process. It also promotes the kind of dangerous growth of fat cells around your vital organs that are the hallmark of diabetes and heart disease. In one study on fructose, 16 volunteers on a controlled diet including high levels of fructose produced new fat cells around their heart, liver and other digestive organs in just 10 weeks![19]

Dr. Mercola goes on to point out that sugar increases leptin and insulin levels and decreases receptor sensitivity for these hormones (known as leptin resistance)—a major factor in premature aging and age-related chronic degenerative diseases. When you eat a typical American diet that is rich in sugar, your blood sugar can elevate and stay that way continually. When you add other refined carbohydrate foods such as bread, cereals, doughnuts, bagels, pasta, pastries, candy, cookies, and sodas, it's easy to see why so many Americans are aging more rapidly than need be.[20]

If nothing else gets your attention, this should. Wrinkles are one aspect of aging that we all try to avoid. When it comes to lines and sagging skin, sugar is your worst enemy. A high-sugar diet damages collagen, the layer just below the skin that gives you that youthful soft appearance. Glycation is what's going on under the surface of the skin of those who look older than they are. As I mentioned before, when you eat sugar, it attaches to proteins to form AGEs. The more sugar you consume, the more AGEs you create. "As AGEs accumulate, they damage adjacent proteins in a domino-like fashion," according to dermatologist Fredric Brandt, MD.[21] According to a study published in the *British Journal of Dermatology*, the effects of aging start around the age of thirty-five. Collagen and elastin keep skin supple and firm, but their protein fibers are the most vulnerable to AGEs damage. So if you want to prevent wrinkles, it's important to protect your collagen. It's the most prevalent protein in your body, but this once springy, resilient protein, like what you had in your twenties, can become dry and brittle. This leads to wrinkles and saggy skin.[22] But it doesn't have to show up with ravaging effects if you eat the right kind of diet, get plenty of vitamin C (which supports collagen), and use good skin care. One of my aunts had beautiful skin with few wrinkles even in her nineties.

A diet that is rich in sugar can also influence the type of collagen your body creates—and this is an important factor in how well your skin is able to resist wrinkles. "The most abundant collagens in the skin are types I, II, and III, with type III being the most stable and longest lasting. Glycation transforms type III collagen into type I, which is more fragile. 'When that happens, the skin looks and feels less supple,' says Brandt."[23] AGEs deactivate the body's antioxidant enzymes, and this leaves your skin highly vulnerable to sun damage—which, in turn, causes skin aging.[24] But the good news about sugar-damaged skin is that it is never too late to stop the cycle. Stop consuming sugar, and rebuild new collagen.

6. Sugar contributes to acid reflux (GERD).

Research shows that a very low-carbohydrate diet improves gastroesophageal reflux (GERD).[25] Another study published in 2008 in the *World Journal of Gastroenterology* found that "GERD is present in about 40% of people with diabetes. The researchers also found GERD to be more common in people with diabetes who also had neuropathy, or nerve damage, which is a common complication of diabetes. People in this study who had diabetes and neuropathy were more likely to have GERD, regardless of weight, compared to people without neuropathy."[26]

For many people, acid reflux is caused by low stomach acid. Common foods that you may eat often, such as doughnuts, cookies, candy, highly preserved foods, sweet sauces and condiments, products baked with white flour, and anything containing high-fructose corn syrup or artificial sweeteners, can lower stomach pH and cause GERD. Many people don't realize that acid reflux is often caused by low stomach acid. That's why drinking 1 to 2 teaspoons apple cider vinegar mixed in 6 ounces of water and taken about fifteen minutes before a meal can help to resolve this problem along with avoiding all sweets and coffee. Highly acidic, coffee can stimulate excessive secretion of gastric acids.

7. Sugar can impair thyroid function.

According to the Association of Clinical Endocrinologists, twenty-seven million Americans are battling with dysfunctional thyroid glands, with many of them going undiagnosed. Another twenty-four million Americans are dealing with subclinical hypothyroidism, a condition in which TSH is elevated but free T4 is normal. Adding these figures together, we see that more than fifty million people in America are affected by some form of thyroid disorder.[27]

SYMPTOMS OF LOW THYROID

- Fatigue
- Weight gain
- Depression
- Constipation
- Hair that falls out easily

- Dry skin
- Poor circulation and numbness in hands and feet
- Morning headaches that wear off as day progresses

If you have impaired thyroid function, you must quit sugar in short order. Sugar can contribute to leaky gut in some individuals, which is often cited as a precursor to an autoimmune disease such as hypothyroidism. Sugar can inflame and muck up your entire endocrine system, which includes the thyroid and adrenal glands. It causes insulin spikes, which harm the thyroid gland and the adrenal glands. In addition to the damage caused by insulin, a compromised thyroid gland will slow the removal of insulin from the bloodstream.

Balancing your blood sugar is critical for healing your thyroid. The body needs a blood sugar range between 70 and 100 milligrams per deciliter (as measured before a meal).[28] Inflammatory chemicals known as cytokines are released in the body when you get out of range. They have a domino effect that is difficult to stop and can lead to thyroid dysfunction.

Blood sugar imbalance and adrenal problems also go hand in hand. If you have one imbalance, you may have the other. This will impact the liver, pituitary gland, gut, heart, and hippocampus. Most of the inactive form of T4 are converted to the active form T3 in the liver. Fluctuations in blood sugar drastically affect the thyroid gland's function in multiple ways. Healing hypothyroidism is futile if your blood sugar level is too high or too low.

To balance your blood sugar, omit all sugar and simple carbohydrates, meaning refined flour products such as bread, rolls, buns, pasta, and pizza. In addition, ditch the alcohol, coffee, soda, junk food, and fast food. Eat plenty of high-fiber vegetables, seeds, nuts, vegetable juices, and green smoothies.[29]

8. Cancer is linked to high levels of sugar in the diet.

Cancer is one of the most feared and deadly diagnoses in our society today. Less than one hundred years ago, in 1931, scientists discovered that cancer cells have a fundamentally different metabolism with regard to energy compared to healthy cells. They learned that malignant tumors exhibit an increase in anaerobic glycolysis—the process in which glucose is converted to fuel by cancer cells, thus creating lactic acid as a by-product. The large amount of lactic acid that is produced in this manner is then transported to the liver and creates a lower, more acidic pH in the cancerous tissues in addition to symptoms of physical fatigue due to the buildup of lactic acid. In other words, they discovered that larger tumors seemed to exhibit a more acidic pH.[30]

In 2004 obesity, diabetes, and cancer were linked by researchers. These researchers learned that you are much more likely to get cancer if you're obese or diabetic—and you're also more likely to get cancer if you have metabolic syndrome.[31] Many different studies around this same time frame have led us to believe that a large percentage of the cancers that we see today are actually caused by our Western diets and lifestyles. The good news is that this means *cancer is actually preventable*, if we would pinpoint the problems and avoid the foods and things that make us sick!

Most cancers and diabetes are relatively rare among people who don't eat Western diets—and in some cases they are virtually nonexistent. Unfortunately, now that we have seen the link between our Western diet and lifestyle and cancer, cancer rates have increased dramatically, especially when obesity and diabetes became more prevalent.[32]

When our bodies develop insulin resistance, we must secrete more insulin to process the sugars in our diet; but unfortunately, insulin, as well as a related hormone known as an insulin-like growth factor, actually promotes tumor growth. Gary Taubes, in his 2011 *New York Times* article, says this:

> The cells of many human cancers come to depend on insulin to provide the fuel (blood sugar) and materials they need to grow and multiply....The more insulin, the better they do. Some cancers develop mutations that serve the purpose of increasing the influence of insulin on the cell; others take advantage of the elevated insulin levels that are common to metabolic syndrome, obesity and type 2 diabetes. Some do both. [Craig Thompson, president of Memorial Sloan-Kettering Cancer Center in New York] believes that many pre-cancerous cells would never acquire the mutations that turn them into malignant tumors if they weren't being driven by insulin to take up more and more blood sugar and metabolize it.[33]

Elevated insulin, especially as seen in an obese or overweight society, often shows up in the development of many cancers, especially in breast and colon cancers. Lewis Cantley, director of the Cancer Center at Beth Israel Deaconess Medical Center at Harvard Medical School, has suggested that 80 percent of human cancers are promoted by mutations of cells and/or environmental factors that enhance the influence of insulin on tumor cells, causing them to grow.[34]

But could it be possible that by avoiding sugar we could suppress insulin's effect on cancer cell growth?

For this very reason, some of the researchers in this study have chosen to avoid sugar or high-fructose corn syrup, if at all possible.

"I have eliminated refined sugar from my diet and eat as little as I possibly can," Thompson said, "because I believe ultimately it's something I can do to decrease my risk of cancer."[35]

Sugar should scare you too. It scares me. My mother died of breast cancer when I was six years old, and she was only forty-four. I learned that her diet was high in sugar and low in vegetables, which she didn't like very much. She had a "sweet tooth" like my grandfather. Unfortunately she never learned the dangers of the treats she loved so much.

9. Sugar contributes to arterial disease.

High levels of blood sugar are extremely damaging to our blood vessels, and the long-term results of arterial disease usually involve heart disease and strokes. This is ultimately caused by sugar consumption.[36] A report from the Nurses' Health Study showed that women who ate diets with a high number of processed sweets and starches had a greatly increased cardiovascular risk.[37] Sugar contributes to inflammation of the arterial walls. Insulin spikes may frequently be caused by high blood sugar. Unfortunately if your insulin spikes on a continual basis, it can damage the fragile endothelial lining of your blood vessels. When this lining is damaged, plaque—made up of cholesterol, fatty substances, cellular waste, calcium, and fibrin (a clotting material in the blood)—will soon form over the injuries, much like a scab forms over a cut. This can, in turn, lead to a blockage of the vessel and eventually a heart attack or a stroke.

According to a report from Tel Aviv University's Sackler School of Medicine and the Heart Institute of Sheba Medical Center, high blood sugar, especially following a meal, has been recognized as a significant risk factor for cardiovascular disease.[38] "Looking inside" the arteries, researcher Michael Shechter says he was able to see that cornflakes and sugar literally caused a stretching and swelling in the arteries *for several hours*, when the person's blood sugar was spiking. While elasticity in the arteries is generally a good thing, when the artery is aggravated over a long period of time, a sudden expansion and then contraction of the arterial wall can reduce its flexibility, promoting heart disease or even a heart attack.[39]

The next time you're tempted to pick up a soda, order a syrupy latte, or drink a sweet iced tea with lunch, think about this research. There is strong evidence that even one sugary beverage per day raises the risk of dying of heart disease by 34 percent.[40]

10. Sugar affects us spiritually.

Many people who have been on my program have said they have realized great spiritual changes when they got off of sugar and changed their diet. Scores of people said their prayer life changed after they omitted sugar. They comprehended spiritual readings with better clarity, and they believed they heard from God more clearly. Why would this be? Is it possible that sugar has an effect on the spirit like it has on the brain? A spiritual fog? Those who have experienced it would say that is true. Your body's desire for food has roots in your soul's need for spiritual intimacy with God. As we grow spiritually, we will see our body as a temple in which our spirit dwells and how much we need to care for it in order to nurture our connection with God.

11. Sugar promotes insomnia.

When you eat sweets, you may not sleep well at all. It has to do with a poorly functioning hypothalamic-pituitary-adrenal axis, and adrenal fatigue or adrenal dysfunction, says Dr. Marsha Nunley, MD. As she states, insomnia is already very common in our stressful, overworked, and burned-out culture. In such an environment, your body's stress hormone, cortisol, produced by the adrenal glands, is overproduced. One function of cortisol is to maintain your body's glucose levels, keeping our brains, hearts, and muscles supplied with glucose, and therefore with energy. Cortisol is therefore essential to life, and your body will produce it when you are stressed—in order to save your life. However, your body does not necessarily know or care the reason that you are stressed. Whether you are running away from a wild animal or you have eaten too much sugar—your body does not know the difference. It will practice the fight-or-flight response no matter the stimulus.[41]

Over the years, as they overproduce cortisol in response to the never-ending modern stressors we face today, your adrenal glands eventually begin to misfire and their signals become erratic. The result is that your blood sugar can get too low or too high because of erratic cortisol, often resulting in sweating, a pounding heart, and an anxious alertness that causes your mind to chatter away in the night.[42]

This is where sugar comes into play. Sweets cause your blood sugar to dip too low, which is usually in the middle of the night. Then you wake up and can't get back to sleep. So, no more ice cream, chocolate, or even fruit in the evening. What about the glass of wine you enjoy in the evening? Grapes are very high in sugar so it might be a villain in disguise as well. You need vegetables and protein. I know people can eat sweets made even with healthy sweetener, and it will affect their sleep for many nights to come. I'm one of those people.

Killing Us Sweetly

Look online for what the establishment has to say about the dangers of sugar. There are as many studies showing there's no problem with sugar as there are studies telling us about the dangers. It's as wild and crazy as a three-year-old after an ice cream party. The sugar lobby is alive and well. Researchers get paid off. Truth-tellers get blacklisted. And the sugar industry continues to produce sugar in all its forms, and food manufacturers continue to dump more and more of it into their products each year, killing us sweetly with their song that all is well because it tastes delicious.

Chapter 4

KNOCK OUT FOGGY SUGAR BRAIN, BAD MOOD, AND DEPRESSION

AVE YOU EVER felt like a morning cloud settled over your brain? It's when you're struggling to remember your coworker's last name or what you agreed to do for your neighbor. It's no fun at all. If you've had a bout of forgetfulness, difficulty thinking, or mental fatigue, you know about brain fog. Maybe you've been riding the blood sugar roller coaster. You eat sweets; your blood sugar spikes. Then it dips low. Well, guess what? Low blood sugar is a known trigger for brain fog symptoms. On top of that poor blood sugar management, (diabetes and hypoglycemia) is known to contribute to cognitive impairment. This is especially true for diabetics, and it can lead to more serious problems such as Alzheimer's disease. A study published in *The Journal of Physiology* found that sugar indeed impairs brain function. If your blood sugar level falls too low, your energy supply to all tissues, and particularly your brain, is impaired. Eating excess sugar, and eating refined carbohydrates, which are rapidly digested into sugar, can overwhelm the body's blood sugar control system.[1]

In premodern times people ate a diet that was low in sugar, and they never had refined carbohydrates. Our modern diet is something new, something the body can't handle. When food is digested, the sugars travel from the gut to the liver, where they are processed. But when you eat sugar or refined carbohydrates, this can overwhelm your liver as sugar floods into the bloodstream. If it's not taken up by the cells, high blood sugar is the result. This affects your brain. If blood sugar levels dip too low, the brain goes into panic mode at the possibility of its fuel supply giving out because it survives on glucose. In response we can get symptoms of hypoglycemia. Then we crave carbs, which will raise blood sugar again! If we don't get them, we feel shaky, weak, and can get a foggy brain. It can become a roller coaster of ups and downs throughout the day.[2]

Is Your Hippocampus Shrinking?

Changes in the size of the hippocampus (memory center) have been correlated with a declining memory. It is interesting to note that blood sugar tests can predict the rate at which the hippocampus will shrink and memory will decline. In a report published in the *Neurology* journal (2013), 141 individuals with an average age of sixty-three years were evaluated regarding memory testing and MRI scans of the brain. The size of the hippocampus of each person was measured along with blood sugar. A correlation was observed between "lower than average blood sugar and better scores in delayed recall, learning ability, and memory consolidation."[3] A correlation was also found between blood sugar and the size of the hippocampus. The researchers stated that "even in the absence of manifest type 2 diabetes mellitus or impaired glucose tolerance, chronically higher blood glucose levels exert a negative influence on cognition, possibly [brought about] by structural changes in learning....Therefore, strategies aimed at lowering glucose levels even in the normal [blood sugar] range may beneficially influence cognition." Their scientific conclusion was that blood sugar is directly associated with brain function and brain structure.[4]

Improve Your Memory and Sidestep Alzheimer's

Today, I came from the assisted-living Alzheimer's and dementia center where we were visiting my husband's stepfather. He has Alzheimer's disease. It's been a steady spiral down that involves loss of brain function, dignity, and quality of life. Yet he is better than many of the people who also reside there, like the cute lady who smiles all the time and makes no sense when she talks, or the much younger woman who has early onset Alzheimer's and is almost completely nonfunctional. Ending up in this state seems to be nearly everyone's greatest fear.

Do you find yourself worried when you forget things, misplace stuff, or just feel fogged in? We joke about our forgetfulness at times—our sunglasses on our heads as we search for them—but the seriousness of the issue is our mental performance and long-term brain health. If forgetfulness and brain fog persists, it can signal the beginning of dementia or Alzheimer's. We can't let that go. We *can* do something about it.

Memory and cognition can be improved, as can the ability to focus mentally and utilize one's mental capacities successfully on demand. Symptoms of poor mental performance include impaired learning ability, poor recall of information, and difficulty following conversation or train of thought.

To improve your memory, you must have adequate nutrition and amino acid balance, and of course, stop eating sugar. It is also important to address allergies, candidiasis, parasites, thyroid disorders, low or high blood sugar, and poor circulation to the brain. General decline in mental performance and actual damage to brain cells and shrinkage of the brain are caused most often by free-radical damage. Free radicals are highly reactive molecules that lack an electron; they attack cells to steal an electron to make themselves stable. In the process, they damage cells. This is the process we want to stop.

Could You Have Brain Sludge?

Damaged cells become free radicals, and a chain reaction is set in motion. The free radicals have gone on a rampage in your body to get electrons. They can attack proteins in the brain. This turns them into "sludge" called lipofuscin—a form of brown slime that can coat neurons. Ronald M. Lawrence, MD, PhD, a specialist in neurology and an assistant clinical professor at UCLA School of Medicine, says, "that slime decreases the ability of the brain to send vital electrochemical messages to other parts of the brain. As the slime thickens, memory declines and senility and dementia begin."[5]

Free-radical damage to the hypothalamus and pituitary glands results in a decline in growth hormone (GH). Low GH can contribute to more of the manifestations of aging, including problems with sleep. Poor sleep further contributes to mental decline. Free-radical attack on the adrenal glands results in a decline in dehydroepiandrosterone (DHEA)—a hormone essential to the ability to learn and form memories.

Due to a host of modern industrial pollutants, processed foods, too many sweets, computers and other sources of low-electromagnetic-field toxicity, and other generators of free radicals, many middle-aged and even younger people are suffering a decline in memory, ability to learn, cognition, intelligence, and the capacity to think clearly. Peak mental performance is a necessity for many people. Business meetings require that you be in top form. There are reports to go over, facts to memorize, and summaries to write. Your job demands an alert, quick mind. If you are a student, school makes great demands on your brain. Also social settings and doing simple tasks, even if you are retired, call for clear thinking. You want to stop any mental decline and get your brain back in top shape.

What is your first step to do so? Scavenge free radicals and prevent attacks on brain cells with an abundance of antioxidant nutrients such as those you find in fresh vegetable juice and wheatgrass juice. As you feed your body high-quality "brain food" every day, you'll see a difference. You have to also remove substances that contribute to brain decline such as all sugars and artificial sweeteners. Artificial sweeteners are neurotoxins that are worse for the brain than sugar. Avoid all junk food as well, which is very bad for the brain.

Whether you want to improve memory or enhance creativity, concentration, or alertness and prevent brain aging, dietary boosters from juicing and nutritional supplements can make a tremendous difference.

The Mood-Brain-Sugar Connection

Sugar can contribute to or exacerbate nervousness, anxiety, and depression. There is a clear link between excess sugar and disorders like anxiety, depression, and schizophrenia. This is due to high levels of insulin and adrenaline that get released with sugar consumption. Some health professionals believe that sugar does not cause anxiety, but others believe that it does. No matter the view, it's been proven that sugar does create changes in various parts of the body that can worsen anxiety or trigger anxiety attacks. Blood sugar imbalance can cause fatigue, distressed thinking, blurry vision, and an overall feeling of illness. Some of the physical symptoms of anxiety, like shaking and nervousness, can be caused by a sugar rush and sugar withdrawal.

Take a look at the mood disorders that studies have linked to sugar. With the increase of sugar in the American diet, it's no wonder that these disorders are on the rise.

- **Increased anxiety.** A study in 2008 found that rats placed on sugar and then deprived of it appeared to have imbalanced dopamine and increased anxiety.[6]

- **Impaired memory and reduced ability to fight anxiety.** In another study it was shown that long-term use of sugar appeared to impair memory and reduce the ability to fight anxiety.[7]

- **Depression.** According to a study in the *American Journal of Clinical Nutrition* (2015), a high-glycemic diet can lead to depression in postmenopausal women.[8] In addition, "the study by James Gangwisch, PhD, and colleagues in the department of psychiatry at Columbia University Medical Center looked at the dietary glycemic index, glycemic load, types of carbohydrates consumed, and depression in data from more than 70,000 postmenopausal women who participated in the National Institutes of Health's Women's Health Initiative Observational Study between 1994 and 1998....Refined foods such as white bread, white rice, and soda trigger a hormonal response in the body to reduce blood sugar levels. This response may also cause or exacerbate mood changes, fatigue, and other symptoms of depression. The investigators found that progressively higher dietary GI [glycemic index] scores and consumption of added sugars and refined grains were associated with increased risk of new-onset depression in postmenopausal women."[9]

Sugar is one of the top contributors to chronic inflammation, which has been implicated in depression. Studies have shown a high rate of depression in countries with high sugar consumption.

Refined sugar and carbohydrates including white bread, refined flour pasta, white rice, and most processed foods are linked with depression. These types of foods require large amounts of B vitamins to turn sugar into energy. *The British Journal of Psychiatry* published a study, which involved 3,500 middle-aged civil servants, found that those who consumed more processed foods had a 58 percent increased risk for depression, and those who ate more whole foods had a 26 percent reduced risk for depression.[10]

Sugar diverts chromium, a trace mineral involved in mood. This mineral is vital in balancing your blood sugar because insulin requires it to operate.[11] According to Dr. Scott Olson, there's another reason sugar sets people up for depression: "Researchers suggest that the sugar and brain association may be due to the oxidative stress that sugar can cause or the change in beta-endorphins (brain chemicals that make us feel good) that comes about because of sugar use."[12] Oxidative degradation of mitochondria in brain cells is also recognized as a major contributor to aging.[13]

- **Schizophrenia.** Talk about sugar shock! Researchers have linked sugar consumption to an increased risk of depression and exacerbation of symptoms in individuals with schizophrenia. Sugar suppresses a key growth hormone in your brain called brain-derived neurotrophic factor (BDNF). In both depression and schizophrenia, BDNF levels are critically low.[14]

- **Irritability, mood swings, brain fog, and fatigue.** There is no doubt that sugar has negative effects on your brain. It interrupts your cognitive function and psychological health. "If you've ever experienced a sugar crash, then you know that sudden peaks and drops in blood sugar levels can cause you to experience symptoms like irritability, mood swings, brain fog and fatigue."[15] When we indulge in something sweet like a cupcake, doughnut, energy bar, or a syrupy latte, it causes blood sugar to spike and then plummet. As your blood sugar dips or crashes, you may experience anxiousness, moodiness, irritability, or depression.[16]

- **Aggressive behavior, anxiety, and depression.** The Brain Bio Center, a nonprofit clinic run by FoodfortheBrain.org, provides nutrition, diet, and lifestyle recommendations to heal mental health conditions. They note that blood sugar imbalances are many times the primary factor in mood disorders.[17] Their article on depression says the following: "Eating lots of sugar is going to give you sudden peaks and troughs in the amount of glucose in your blood; symptoms that this is going on include fatigue, irritability, dizziness, insomnia, excessive sweating (especially at night), poor concentration and forgetfulness, excessive thirst, depression and crying spells, digestive disturbances and blurred vision. Since the brain depends on an even supply of glucose it is no surprise to find that sugar has been implicated in aggressive behavior, anxiety, and depression, and fatigue."[18]

- **Schizophrenia and depression.** Malcolm Peet, a noted British psychiatric researcher, has found a link between sugar and both depression and schizophrenia.[19] Animals demonstrating the highest ability to learn spatial and memory tasks also had the most BDNF. But two months on a high-sugar diet significantly reduced BDNF in the brains of the animals. This had an effect on their ability to perform spatial and memory tasks.[20] "Low BDNF is no small thing, as it has also been associated with depression, obsessive-compulsive disorder, Alzheimer's disease and other dementias, Huntington's disease, Rett syndrome, and schizophrenia....But there is much more to the sugar-brain story than BDNF."[21] "There are quite a few clinical studies that link the consumption of grains (foods that act like sugar) with schizophrenia."[22]

The Brain-Boosting, Mood-Enhancing Diet

How we think has a lot to do with how we eat. In fact, diet is extremely important. According to Dr. Lawrence, "Tests with animals have shown that by withholding certain nutrients from their diets, the animals forgot tricks they had learned or could not find their way out of a maze which they had easily traversed many times before their diet was changed."[23]

Eating a whole foods, clean diet has been shown to improve mental performance and cognitive function. For example, a number of studies have confirmed that school breakfast programs have a positive effect on helping disadvantaged children learn.[24] This leads us to contemplate what happens to the brain with the typical morning cup of coffee and doughnut or toast.

Here's what you can do:

1. Eat a high-fiber, healthy-fat diet. An all-carbohydrate meal, such as an all-fruit or fruit and yogurt breakfast, can adversely affect memory. For best mental performance, combine complex carbohydrates (vegetables; ancient grains such as quinoa, millet, teff, and buckwheat; legumes) with about 10 to 15 percent protein and 15 to 25 percent healthy and essential fatty acids. Essential fatty acids (primarily the omega 3 fatty acids) can help improve mental functions.

2. Avoid refined sugars and alcohol; they "turn off" the brain and contribute to lipofuscin (brain sludge).

3. Juicing and juice fasting help the body get rid of brain sludge (lipofuscin) and prevent free-radical attacks on brain cells due to the high levels of antioxidants. Fresh juices are loaded with antioxidants that bind to the "wild bullet" molecules known as free radicals so that they cannot damage your brain. Juice fasting for several days gives the body a chance to do a thorough "spring cleanup" on the brain. Many people who attend our juice and raw foods retreats

say that after our three-day juice fast, they feel much more alert and alive. They can think more clearly, and their foggy brain flew out the window!

Super Mind Nutrients

Dr. Lawrence says that "many scientists believe that by the age of 60, your body is absorbing an estimated one-third less nutrients from food than a twenty-year-old. So, what does that have to do with your memory? A lot, according to scientists. They have found that your brain needs a daily supply of 15 different nutrients in order to operate efficiently. A shortage of any one of those nutrients can affect your memory and mental ability."[25]

Some tests have shown that certain nutrients will improve cognitive functions. Research shows that a deficiency of certain nutrients can cause memory and learning problems. Supplying the right nutrients can stop a decline in mental function, as well as improve overall mental performance.

The brain uses substances called neurotransmitters to draw memories to your conscious mind. These neurotransmitters—such as acetylcholine (ACh), epinephrine, and serotonin—are electro-chemical messengers that stimulate your memory. You can improve neurotransmitter status with nutrients that support them. Overall brain function can be enhanced by consuming a generous supply of nutrients that empower brain functions and protect the brain from free-radical damage.

- **Choline:** Acetylcholine is an important neurotransmitter for memory and intelligence. It is made from choline, one of the B vitamins. Some studies show that choline significantly improved memory in healthy young adults. When it comes to stress, choline has demonstrated an immediate boost in brainpower. It can also strengthen neurons in the brain's memory centers, thus improving mental functioning and thought processes. It can also slow down age-related loss of dendrites. Choline is found in highest quantities in lecithin. (Lecithin capsules and granules can be purchased at most health food stores.) Best juice sources: green beans, cabbage, spinach, and oranges.

- **Vitamin C:** This potent, cognitive-enhancing antioxidant can boost brainpower. One study has shown vitamin C supplementation, given to those with low levels of this vitamin, increased IQ scores by more than 3.5 points.[26] Best juice sources: bell peppers, kale, parsley, broccoli, brussels sprouts, cauliflower, cabbage, strawberries, papayas, spinach, citrus fruits, mangos, and cantaloupe.

- **Boron:** A trace mineral that has yet to be recognized as essential for human beings, boron deficiencies have been noted to affect cognitive performance. A set of three studies found that low intake of boron resulted in significantly poorer performance on tasks involving encoding, short-term memory, and attention.[27] Fruits and vegetables are the best sources of boron; therefore, you have a wide variety from which to choose.

- **Glutathione:** This is a brain-enhancing substance that increases the flow of blood and oxygen to the brain. It has a protective effect on the brain's cells and boosts mental functions. Best juice sources: asparagus, watermelon, citrus fruits, strawberries, peaches, cauliflower, broccoli, tomatoes, and avocados (avocados don't juice well, but they make a great green smoothie and do well in raw soups).

- **Other brain boosters:** A number of amino acids such as glutamine, phenylalanine, pyrogluta-mate, methionine, and threonine have been shown to enhance learning and memory. Other substances such as N-acetyl-L-carnitine and dimethylglycine (DMG) may also be helpful.

Fight the Good Fight for Your Brain

The good news is that you can change your brain health with the right diet and supplements! When you knock out the sugar, eat a whole foods diet, and add in the brain-boosting nutrients to your diet, you can improve your memory and mood.

Chapter 5

DIABETES, HYPOGLYCEMIA, AND BLOOD SUGAR IMBALANCES: DOWN FOR THE COUNT

D ID YOU KNOW that you can control your blood sugar and heal your body with the right diet, even if you are diabetic, prediabetic, or hypoglycemic? It starts with ditching sugar in all its forms, avoiding all refined carbs, minimizing starchy vegetables, juicing lots of green vegetables, and eating adequate amounts of clean protein. You can bring healing to your pancreas and indeed your whole body.

What is your blood sugar number? The ideal number for healthy non-diabetic people lies between 70 and 99 mg/dl (milligrams of glucose for every deciliter of blood) when fasting, or 90 and 110 mg/dl two hours after eating.[1] But there's another number that is alarming—29 million. That's the number of Americans who are currently diagnosed with diabetes.[2] It is estimated that there are another 8 million who are in the dark about their condition, undiagnosed and unaware of their disease.[3] There are 86 million prediabetics.[4] The incidence of new-onset diabetes in US adults has increased by 90 percent over the past ten years.[5] It costs the United States $245 billion annually. Globally 371 million individuals suffer from diabetes, with 4.8 million who die of the disease each year.[6]

"The odds of developing diabetes increased by 40% from the

1970s to the 1980s and then doubled between the 1970s and 1990s. Analysis by gender revealed an 84% increase in diabetes incidence among women during the 1990s compared with the 1970s. In men, diabetes more than doubled during the 1990s compared with the 1970s."[7]

What changed in the American diet during this time? Sugar. Along came the fat scare in the seventies. Cholesterol and fat were targeted as the cause of the rising incidence of heart disease. Scientists and health professionals sounded the alarm. We were told to get rid of all fats in our diet. In the late 1980s reports identified eating less fat as the single most important change that needed to be made in order to improve health and prevent heart attacks. But fat adds flavor. Take it away and food tastes rather bland. Ah, sugar to the rescue! The food industry obliged and began substituting sugar for fat in almost everything. People looked at labels in terms of fat. If it said "low fat," it was considered good for you. It was kind of like wearing a nutritional seat belt. No one looked for sugar. Sugar is addictive—indeed, it's a drug-like substance—so people wanted more and more of it. Food manufacturers stepped up production. Everyone was happy, at least for a while. But with all the fat-free and low-fat products, Americans got fatter and sicker. Diabetes spiked up. It rose with the increased sugar consumption.

Without fat we experience sugar cravings and frequent hunger. This happens because fat provides satiation after a meal, while carbohydrates alone do not. With the added carbs comes elevated blood sugar. With America's blood sugar skyrocketing and diabetes statistics spiking, you would think health professionals would have seriously looked for the cause. However, except for a few lone voices, no one talked about cause and effect. People have eaten fat for centuries, but never in history had people eaten so much sugar. Very few scientists or health professionals took a look at this fact.

BLOOD SUGAR 101

In order to maintain a healthy blood sugar balance, it is important to understand how it all works. Following are some basic terms used in association with blood sugar:

- Glucose is the body's preferred source of fuel.

- Insulin is a hormone secreted by the pancreas that shuttles glucose to the cells. Insulin rings the doorbell and tells the cells to open up. Its job is to deliver glucose into cells so it can be used for energy.

- Insulin resistance is a failure of the cell door to open to receive the glucose that the insulin wants to shuttle in. When you consume too many refined carbs in the form of sugar and refined grains, blood sugar shoots up. The pancreas goes into action and overcompensates with extra insulin release. This excessive reaction eventually causes insulin resistance, and can lead to type 2 diabetes if a high carb/high sugar diet is continued. However, it can be reversed through a healthy diet that omits sugar and refined carbs to balance your blood sugar.

- Glycogen is a primary storage form of glucose in cells. The liver converts any glucose that doesn't get into the cells into glycogen and stores it until it is needed to stabilize blood sugar between meals and overnight. Stress and hormone imbalances can deplete the body's ability to store glycogen, which in turn contributes to blood sugar imbalance.

- Hyperglycemia is another term for chronically high blood sugar, which can lead to diabetes.

- Hypoglycemia is low blood sugar. Though glycogen should prevent hypoglycemia, when there is an imbalance in your body caused by stress and hormonal imbalances, you can end up with low blood sugar. Usually it happens when you eat a high-carb food and excessive insulin pushes too much sugar into the cells, causing blood sugar to drop too low.

Sugar Versus Glucose

The phrase Dr. Robert Lustig uses when he describes sugar versus glucose is "'isocaloric but not isometabolic.' This means we can eat 100 calories of glucose (from a potato or bread or other starch) or 100 calories of sugar (half glucose and half fructose), and they will be metabolized differently and have a different effect on the body. The calories are the same, but the metabolic consequences are quite different."[8]

Studies conducted upon rats and mice have demonstrated that when fructose reaches the liver in sufficient amounts and with rapid enough speed—in much the same way as when we drink fruit juice or soda—the liver converts most of it to fat. This in turn causes insulin resistance, which has been identified as a strong precursor to type 2 diabetes and is believed to be one underlying cause of many cancers.[9]

Sugar and the Pancreas

Known as a gland, the pancreas is about the size of a small hand, and is situated between a bend in the duodenum (part of the intestines) and the stomach. Though it's small, it has big work to do. It is the body's master chemist, releasing hormones that control blood sugar such as glucagon and insulin. Glucagon stimulates the liver to metabolize glycogen into glucose and raises blood sugar. Other pancreatic hormones, including polypeptide and somatostatin, play a part in regulating and fine-tuning the insulin- and glucagon-producing cells. Too much sugar upsets the delicate balance of this process and cause poor pancreatic function. Symptoms include high blood glucose after eating sugar and carbohydrates, diabetes, metabolic syndrome, and hypoglycemia. If the pancreas is severely affected, a person may also experience vitamin and other nutrient deficiencies.

Sugar can stress the pancreas beyond what it is equipped to deal with. Sugar breaks down quickly in the digestive system. In short order, your bloodstream is flooded with glucose. Then the pancreas releases insulin into the bloodstream to deal with the sugar. Eating too many sweets puts a lot of stress on your pancreas, causing it to age more rapidly. This can result in pancreatic distress such as diabetes, prediabetes, or hypoglycemia.

Does Sugar Cause Diabetes?

A defense attorney might call the correlation between sugar and diabetes "circumstantial evidence." As sugar consumption has risen in this country, there has also been a rise in diabetes.

Frederick Banting, who shared the 1923 Nobel Prize for the discovery of insulin, had the idea that sugar causes diabetes. Banting's theory was "based on the observation that the disease was rare in populations that didn't consume refined sugar and widespread in those that did."[10]

According to one article entitled "Is Sugar Toxic?" in the *New York Times*: "In 1924, Haven Emerson, director of the institute of public health at Columbia University, reported that diabetes deaths in New York City had increased as much as 15-fold since the Civil War years, and that deaths increased as much as fourfold in some U.S. cities between 1900 and 1920."[11] He observed that the rise in diabetes coincided with the increase in sugar consumption (primarily candy and soft drinks during this time), which had nearly doubled between 1890 and the early 1920s.[12]

Elliott Joslin, a pioneering authority on diabetes, attempted to correlate the high white rice diet in Japan with sugar consumption in America. He pointed to the fact that the Japanese eat lots of rice, and Japanese diabetics are few in number. He based his comparison on the fact that rice is mostly carbohydrates, and suggested that sugar, which is also a carbohydrate, does not cause diabetes. However, rice and sugar do not act the same way in the body, and it is faulty thinking to conclude that they do just because they are both carbohydrates. It is the fructose element of the sugar that affects how we metabolize sugar, which is very different from the carbohydrate (starch) of white rice. But Joslin argued his point that sugar played no role in diabetes in each edition of his textbooks, and it eventually became undisputed truth.[13] Until now, that is.

What Causes Hypoglycemia?

The two most significant factors regarding hypoglycemia are diet and stress. The typical American diet, which is high in sugar and refined grains, sodas, sugary drinks, and coffee, is a sure prescription for hypoglycemia. Sugar is absorbed very quickly into the bloodstream because it requires very little digestion. This causes a rapid increase in blood glucose levels, and the pancreas becomes hypersensitive to sugar. As time goes on, the pancreas becomes conditioned to secrete large amounts of insulin as a response to the increase in blood glucose. This quickly lowers blood sugar, which usually falls below normal levels. It is during the low blood sugar period that hypoglycemia symptoms manifest, triggered by a deficiency of glucose to the brain and a corresponding adrenal stress response. (A high carbohydrate diet is one path to adrenal exhaustion.) The more you crave sweets and refined carbs, the more you eat, and the cycle starts over again.

SYMPTOMS OF HYPOGLYCEMIA

- Nervousness
- Irritability
- Emotional problems
- Fatigue
- Depression
- Anxiety
- Cravings for sweets
- Foggy brain
- Inability to concentrate
- Hot and cold sweats
- Shakes
- Heart palpitations
- Tingling of the skin and scalp
- Dizziness/vertigo
- Trembling
- Fainting
- Blurred vision
- Cold hands and feet
- Nausea
- Midmorning and mid-to-late-afternoon tiredness/sleepiness
- Feeling overwhelmed
- Indecisiveness
- Crying spells
- Allergies
- Hyperactivity

Eating lots of carbs causes the pancreas to pump out extra insulin to shuttle all the excess glucose in the bloodstream to the cells to be used for energy. Over time this causes the cells to lose the ability to respond to all of that insulin. It's as if insulin is ringing the doorbell and saying, "Open up!" but the cells can't hear it any longer. There have been too many doorbells, and they are desensitized. The pancreas responds by pumping out more insulin (louder doorbells!) to get glucose into the cells, which causes insulin resistance, and you end up with hypoglycemia symptoms.

You can control hypoglycemia with the right diet. You don't have to experience those nasty symptoms again, unless you go back to your old diet. Then they will come back. I know. I was diagnosed with hypoglycemia in my twenties. That was the era when they diagnosed with the glucose tolerance test where patients were given a glass of thick sugary water that was more like syrup on an empty stomach in the morning after fasting. The test started at 8:00 a.m., and by 10:00 a.m. I had nearly passed out. I was lying on the floor in one of the doctor's office rooms. Needless to say I was diagnosed as hypoglycemic.

Some conventional doctors said a person should have some orange juice or candy if their blood sugar dipped low and they manifested hypoglycemic symptoms. I found that was the worst thing to do. It was far better to cut out all sweets and refined carbs. I had to even cut out fruit except for lemon and lime. No coffee or black tea. I discovered it was very important to eat protein and vegetables. Juicing vegetables made a huge difference in how I felt. This program worked for me and many other people that I've worked with as their nutritionist. I believe it will work for you as well.

Insulin Resistance

Insulin resistance indicates that your cells are ignoring insulin. The body secretes insulin in response to the foods you eat, particularly carbohydrates. Insulin balances your blood sugar after you eat. But when cells become resistant to insulin, blood sugar goes up. The pancreas responds to rising blood sugar by pumping out more and more insulin. For people who keep eating sugar and refined carbohydrates, eventually the pancreas can't keep up with the demand. The person experiences "pancreatic exhaustion." At that point blood sugar rises out of control, and you've got insulin resistance, which can lead to metabolic syndrome or diabetes. Not everyone with insulin resistance gets metabolic syndrome or becomes diabetic. Some people continue to produce enough insulin to overcome their cells' resistance to it. However, this is not a good scenario because chronically elevated insulin levels have harmful effects on the heart and can lead to heart disease.

Metabolic Syndrome

Americans keep getting fatter, and more of them are getting metabolic syndrome. In fact, roughly seventy-five million Americans have metabolic syndrome, according to an estimate from the Centers for Disease Control and Prevention.[14] Physicians have acknowledged that metabolic syndrome is a huge risk factor for diabetes and heart disease. It's is a major reason people have heart attacks.

High blood sugar can cause higher triglyceride levels and blood pressure, lower levels of HDL cholesterol, and increased insulin resistance. This is metabolic syndrome. It could also be called *excess carbohydrate disease* because it is caused by chronic high blood sugar (hyperglycemia). Chronic hyperglycemia is caused by eating too many carbohydrates—sweets and refined carbs.

The first symptom doctors look for in diagnosing metabolic syndrome is an expanding waistline. Everyone who is overweight has a good chance of getting metabolic syndrome, which means that they are more likely to become diabetic or have a heart attack than someone who is not overweight. Trim people can also have metabolic syndrome and be at higher risk of heart disease and diabetes than lean people who don't have it.

Metabolic syndrome affects 50 million Americans, and insulin resistance is one major component, affecting up to 105 million Americans! This problem has increased to the point that it's been predicted to ultimately bankrupt our health-care system.[15] A correlation has also been found between thyroid disorder and metabolic syndrome. An increased frequency of thyroid disorders has also been reported in diabetics.[16] Additionally people with thyroid disorders have much more incidence of obesity and metabolic syndrome, because healthy thyroid function is completely dependent on having a normal blood sugar level. It is so important to keep your blood sugar in normal range! Continual insulin spikes, such as what people experience when they have insulin resistance, can damage the thyroid gland. When the thyroid gland is impaired, thyroid hormone production falls.

To best assess the risk of heart disease, it's important to look at LDL cholesterol particles (the bad cholesterol), inflammation markers, and symptoms of metabolic syndrome. According to Gary Taubes's article, "Scott Grundy, a University of Texas Southwestern Medical Center nutritionist and the chairman of the panel that produced the last edition of the National Cholesterol Education Program guidelines, [says] that heart attacks 50 years ago might have been caused by high cholesterol—particularly high LDL cholesterol—but since then we've all gotten fatter and more diabetic, so now it's metabolic syndrome that is the more conspicuous problem."[17]

Researchers think it is fat in the liver that sets off insulin resistance. "Varman Samuel, who studies insulin resistance at

Yale School of Medicine, [says] the correlation between liver fat and insulin resistance in patients, lean or obese, is 'remarkably strong.'"[18] It is assumed that when people gain weight, it leads to a fatty liver, but this does not explain why lean people get a fatty liver. Rather than weight gain, metabolic syndrome is more likely caused by consuming sugar. "If you want to cause insulin resistance in laboratory rats, says Gerald Reaven, the Stanford University diabetologist...feeding them diets that are mostly fructose is an easy way to do it. It's a 'very obvious, very dramatic' effect."[19] The researchers found that when animals are fed pure fructose or sugar, their livers convert those substances into fat, which is linked with heart disease.[20]

METABOLIC SYNDROME RISK FACTORS

- Excess abdominal weight
- High cholesterol and triglycerides
- High blood pressure
- Insulin resistance
- Tendency to form blood clots
- Inflammation

You Can Heal Insulin Resistance and Metabolic Syndrome

Stop eating sweets and refined carbs. That's right—it's that simple. You can heal these sugar imbalances. Colorado State University biochemist Michael Pagliassotti conducted numerous animal studies in the late 1990s. Pagliassotti says that "changes can happen in as little as a week if the animals are fed sugar or fructose in huge amounts—60 or 70 percent of the calories in their diets. They can take several months if the animals are fed [a diet] closer to what humans (in America) actually consume—around 20 percent of the calories in their diet."[21] He found that when researchers stopped feeding the animals sugar, the fatty liver went away, and so did the insulin resistance.[22]

Get Healthy: The Diet for Diabetes, Hypoglycemia, Insulin Resistance, and Metabolic Syndrome

High blood sugar (diabetes and prediabetes) is only one of the sugar balance disorders facing people today. In type 1 diabetes the pancreas completely loses its ability to produce insulin. In type 2 diabetes the cells of the body partially or fully lose their ability to use insulin (insulin resistance). Metabolic syndrome (insulin resistance) and hypoglycemia (low blood sugar) also plague a large percentage of people. Whatever blood sugar issue you have been diagnosed with, you can heal your body and balance your blood sugar by choosing the right diet, supplements, and lifestyle. It's important to consume healthy sources of carbohydrates, such as vegetables and vegetable juices with limited whole grains, and with plenty of healthy fats and clean protein.

This style of eating allows glucose from a meal to enter your bloodstream slowly. It also supports the pancreas to respond appropriately by secreting smaller amounts of insulin. This assists insulin in transporting the right portion of glucose into cells to be used for energy. This prevents excess insulin from floating through your bloodstream and promoting inflammation. When you balance blood sugar throughout the day, you will keep insulin under control and your blood sugar levels stable. When you eat the right diet, you should be able to go without food for three or four hours between snacks and meals without experiencing blood sugar imbalance symptoms such as sugar cravings or feeling shaky, irritable, or tired. Blood sugar imbalances stoke inflammation, whereas stable blood sugar reduces inflammation and balances hormones. Get your blood sugar in balance, and say good-bye to sugar cravings. Then you can watch stubborn weight melt away along with a crabby mood, foggy brain, dizziness, and weakness.

It's time to get started on a lifestyle that offers a healthier, happier you. Though it may seem at first that you are deprived of eating pleasure, what you will have in the end is a healthier body, and that's true pleasure—the kind that lasts a lifetime.

You Can Control Diabetes and Other Blood Sugar Disorders With Diet

1. No sugar. Cutting out sweets is the most important step you can take in balancing your blood sugar. In plain English: you've got to stop eating *all* sweets. It's the only way you'll get balanced blood sugar and stay well. I've heard many protests. You may be thinking of some right now. But the only way to have the health you want is to let go of what is making you sick. Sugar comes in many forms, so read labels and ditch it all. (For the sweetener shopping guide, see chapter 8.)

2. No artificial sweeteners. This means sucralose (Splenda), aspartame (NutraSweet, Equal), acesulfame potassium (Sunett, Sweet One), and saccharin (Sugar Twin, Sweet'N Low). Though these sweetener substitutes are advertised as zero calories and are not

supposed to raise your blood sugar, they are worse for your body than actual sugar. They are not a good alternative for diabetics, and they are more fattening than sugar. See chapter 8 for more information.

3. No energy bars or low-glycemic bars. They are all sweetened with some form of sweetener. They have sweeteners like mannitol, which is a sugar alcohol, and are not low glycemic.

4. No diet sodas or regular sodas. Don't even drink the ones sweetened with stevia. They use too much stevia.

5. Eat high-quality fat with carbohydrates. Whenever you eat carbohydrates, they should be accompanied with "good fat." Good fat is the kind that slows down the release of glucose into the bloodstream and it will prevent the sugar highs and lows in your blood. Fat also makes us feel satiated, that feeling of satisfaction after we eat that tells us to stop consuming food. Fat makes us feel full longer so that we ultimately snack less, and that helps us lose weight. And finally fat prompts the gallbladder to release bile. If you follow a low-fat diet for a while, bile can become thick and stagnant. Bile transports toxins released from the liver that should leave the body, but stagnant bile unfortunately holds on to toxins like carcinogens, chemicals, pharmaceuticals, and heavy metals, which give them the opportunity to be reabsorbed back into the body. If that happens we experience inflammation and toxic overload. Extra-virgin olive oil, virgin coconut oil, grape seed oil, flax seeds, and

avocado are excellent fat choices to incorporate into your meals.

6. Smaller, more frequent meals or larger, less frequent meals? Which is better? There are health scientists on both sides of this issue with their reasons why each is good. You must decide what works for you. It may be necessary for you to eat more frequent meals if you have an autoimmune disease, adrenal fatigue, chronic fatigue, inflammation, low thyroid, low blood sugar, or poor digestion. If your blood sugar balance can be maintained, short intermittent fasts may be healthful for these conditions.

7. Eat breakfast and include some fat and protein. It is important to balance your blood sugar in the morning by eating breakfast within thirty to forty-five minutes of awakening. You have just fasted for the night, unless you have nocturnal hypoglycemia and you've been up scavenging for food in the night. If you are not hungry for breakfast or the thought of food makes you nauseous in the morning, it may indicate that you have slow digestion due to low stomach acid. If this is the case, you should take HCL Betaine (1 to 3 capsules) in the middle of each meal. It can also indicate that your stress hormones are out of balance. When you skip breakfast, your stress hormones increase and begin to break down muscle instead of fat. This stresses out your body and messes up your blood sugar for the day.

You should include clean proteins, healthy fat, and

a source of carbohydrates such as a juice combination that has a variety of vegetables. You could drink a vegetable juice followed by a green smoothie made with avocado and sprinkle some seeds or chopped nuts on top. Or you could sauté vegetables with eggs. Include ground flaxseeds often; they are tied to decreased insulin resistance.

8. Eat protein. Protein helps in the process of shuttling glucose into the cells so your body can use it for energy. Protein snacks can help keep your blood sugar balanced. Our macronutrients—fats, proteins, and carbohydrates—all work together. We have problems when we deviate from a healthy plan with either poor-quality macronutrients or eating them out of proportion. For example, an all-fruit or fruit and yogurt breakfast could send your blood sugar into outer space and you'll end up spacey all morning.

9. Ditch most protein powders. For the most part, they are not the healthiest choices. In a pinch, plant-based protein powders can give you a little boost, but they should not be relied on for protein in the morning all the time (like in the morning smoothie). And most of them have sweeteners. However, a green smoothie with avocado, powdered greens like barley grass and wheatgrass, and some nuts or seeds is a good choice.

10. Watch the grains. Yes, indeed, we need to turn the pyramid upside down. A gluten-free diet is the new fad, but that's not enough. I recommend going gluten-free due to the genetic composition of modern wheat

(hybridizing to get more gluten for fluffier bread) and the methods of wheat production, including the use of pesticides sprayed right on the grain to ripen it quickly. However, a gluten-free diet does not automatically help you avoid all the grains that turn to sugar easily, and gluten-free products often include inflammatory ingredients like polyunsaturated vegetable oils, soy, and sugar. "Healthy whole grains" are not particularly healthy for your blood sugar. When ground into flour, most grains act like sugar in the body, triggering weight gain, inflammation, and blood-sugar imbalances. We're confronted with gluten in all its tantalizing forms—toast, bagels, cereal, crackers, pancakes, sandwiches, wraps, pasta, pizza, and the restaurant bread basket. All of this turns to sugar. It doesn't matter whether it's brown bread, wheat bread, or a whole grain muffin. If it has flour, it will turn to sugar quickly. It's time to clean it all out of the pantry, freezer, and fridge. And ditch all the flour products. You can have some ancient, whole grains, such as old-fashioned oats, quinoa, teff, kamut, buckwheat, millet, and amaranth.

11. Choose complex carbohydrates that include vegetables and low-sugar fruits. Complex carbohydrates like vegetables provide your body with the preferred source of fuel—glucose. Enjoy low-sugar fruit such as green apples, berries, lemons, and limes. All vegetables are excellent. Root vegetables such as sweet potatoes, carrots, celeriac, and beets can help you satisfy a sweet tooth. For the first thirty days, avoid

white potatoes. Make healthy vegetable juices. You can flavor them with some lemon or lime, ginger (an anti-inflammatory), and a little green apple. Keep the carrots and beets low since they are high-sugar vegetables. People often say they can't juice because their doctor said it's too high in sugar. Yes, fruit juice is too high in sugar. But vegetable juice is not. Diabetics can juice vegetables with an emphasis on the green veggies. Juicing green beans is especially good for the pancreas; mix it with other great-tasting veggies.

12. Get quality sleep. Did you once sleep like a champ but not today? Sleep deprivation wreaks havoc on your blood sugar. Do you need to improve your sleep? This will support healthy blood sugar levels. Sleep deprivation affects blood sugar in numerous ways. Research indicates that a lack of sleep can impair your body's ability to metabolize glucose. This increases insulin production, which leads to an increased risk of diabetes.

Sleep deprivation also causes imbalances of the hormones that regulate your appetite: leptin and ghrelin. As you might imagine, when these hormones are out of balance, you are likely to eat more and gain weight.[23] Inadequate sleep also reduces glucose tolerance, making it more difficult for cells to take in glucose and creating higher blood sugar. One study found that "less than 1 week of sleep restriction can result in a prediabetic state in young, healthy subjects."[24] If you have tried various sleep remedies and nothing has worked, you may need to balance your brain neurotransmitters.

13. Exercise. Include moderate exercise, such as walking, in your healthy living plan. Exercise makes your heart beat a little faster. Your muscles use more glucose, thus pulling more sugar from your bloodstream. This helps to balance your blood sugar levels and improve the body's use of insulin for hours. To reap the most benefit, stick to moderate activity. A more intense workout can temporarily increase your blood sugar levels after you stop exercising, and a really strenuous workout can signal your body to create stress hormones and actually raise your blood sugar.

Supplements to Help Balance Blood Sugar

1. Berberine (goldenseal) in its hydrochloride form has been used to treat diabetes and cardiovascular dysfunction. It works on the insulin receptor, increasing the cell's glucose consumption. It also is helpful for the cardiovascular system, lipids, and liver. It is an effective hypoglycemia agent. Prescription drugs for diabetics can have a variety of adverse effects, including liver problems. Berberine lowers elevated liver enzymes. It is very good for diabetics with liver problems.

2. Common ash can help balance blood sugar. The liver stores sugar as glycogen. Between meals and at night the liver turns glycogen into glucose, but an overburdened liver becomes less efficient at this regulation,

especially for those with fatty liver disease. That's where common ash comes in. It aids the liver in handling sugar. The seeds of this plant appear to inhibit the reabsorption of glucose.

3. Silymarin (milk thistle) regulates glucose and protects against related liver and cardiac dysfunction.

4. Chromium picolinate combined with biotin is known to improve glucose regulation.

5. Magnesium citrate plays an important role in insulin sensitivity and homeostasis.

Juice Recipes for Diabetes and Other Blood Sugar Problems

If you have blood sugar metabolism problems, it is best to avoid fruit. Juice vegetables instead. You may also need to minimize carrots and beets, as they are the vegetables with the highest levels of sugar. You may be able to add one-half of an apple, but make it a green apple, which is lower in sugar. As a nutritionist I've worked with a number of diabetics, hypoglycemics, and other people with blood sugar metabolism problems who have been able to control their blood sugar by changing their diets to the one presented in my book *The Juice Lady's Anti-Inflammation Diet* and by juicing their vegetables.

Following are several recipes:

Pancreas Helper Cocktail

1 large vine-ripened tomato
8 organic string beans
½ small or medium lemon, peeled

Cut produce to fit your juicer's feed tube. Juice ingredients and stir. Drink as soon as possible. Serves 1.

Note: Green beans are known to be good for the pancreas.

The Blood Sugar–Balancing Cocktail

2 romaine lettuce leaves
1 cucumber, peeled
1 celery rib
1 carrot (optional)
8–10 string beans
2 brussels sprouts
½ lemon, peeled
1 tomato

Bunch up romaine lettuce leaves. Cut produce to fit your juicer's feed tube. Tuck the romaine lettuce in the feed tube and push through with the cucumber. Juice remaining ingredients, finishing with some tomato. Pour into a glass and drink as soon as possible. Serves 1.

Note: brussels sprouts and string bean juice have been used as traditional remedies to help strengthen and support the pancreas. For best pancreas support, also avoid refined carbohydrates such as white flour products, sugars of all type, soda, and all sweets. Drink before a meal. (If this drink is too strong, dilute with a little water.)

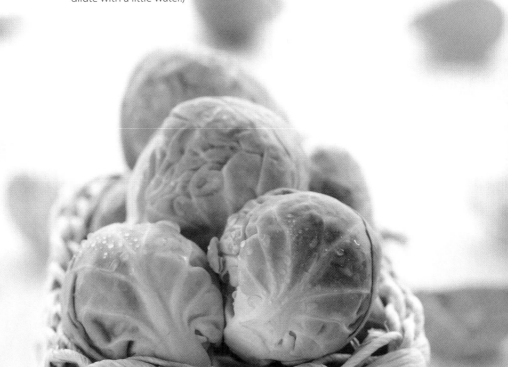

Healing Your Body One Meal at a Time

As you make mealtime changes and healthy choices to balance your blood sugar, your health will improve. Make sure to increase healthy fat and protein at your meals and decrease the refined and starchy carbs. Ditch sugar for good. You may need to avoid all fruit for a while as you learn to tweak your diet to get results. If your blood sugar is too low between meals, consider increasing the protein and complex carbs, and include a snack, such as seeds or nuts. You'll be on your way to balanced blood sugar in short order.

Chapter 6

TAKING OFF THE GLOVES: HOW TO STRENGTHEN YOUR IMMUNE SYSTEM

S TRENGTHENING AND MAINTAINING your immune system is tantamount to good health because it is your first line of defense against disease. Every part of your immune system— your thymus, spleen, adenoids, tonsils, lymph nodes, white blood cells, and more—works together to protect your body from foreign invaders that threaten your body with infection and disease.

Environmental toxins (pollution, pesticides, cigarette smoke), free radicals, pathogens (yeasts, fungi, parasites), stress, poor dietary habits including too many simple carbohydrates, nutrient deficiencies (including subclinical), overuse of antibiotics, and poor digestion all contribute to a weakened immune system. When immunity is down the body ages faster and problems such as cancer cells, infections, and illnesses have a greater chance of developing "under the radar."

Research with rats has shown that sucralose (Splenda) caused the thymus gland to shrink up to 40 percent when consumed in large doses.[1] The thymus gland is the major gland of the immune system, so this could present a real problem. Free radicals also attack immune cells. (Free radicals are unstable molecules that lack an electron and are constantly attacking other cells to steal one of those little guys. This rampage sets up a chain reaction creating large numbers of damaged cells.) Signs of a weakened immune system include more than one cold or flu a year, viruses, infections, and other more serious illnesses such as cancer.

Contacting germs is natural. The world around us is populated with trillions of them. Every time you inhale, sip water, and eat food, you get a dose of germs. We are all vulnerable to attacks by them. So what makes one person sick while others stay healthy under the same conditions? It's the strength of the immune system. A strong immune system fights against germs and keeps you in the pink of health. People who have a weak immune system catch illnesses such as colds, flu, and bronchitis more easily.

In order to boost your immune system and decrease your odds of developing disease, review all elements of your lifestyle that might need improvement. Because the body is quite adaptable, we are able to eat poor foods and still manage to get by while we live an unhealthy lifestyle for years. We may even appear healthy. But sooner or later, it catches up with us. For me it was sooner than later. We are told that to stay healthy we need to eat a balanced diet, but "balance" to some people means balancing one processed food, fast-food item, or junk food with another. Instead we should eat a nutrient-rich diet, drink eight glasses of pure water each day, get regular exercise, and keep a positive attitude.

Sugar Compromises the Immune System

Have you ever wondered why so many people get sick in January and February? Could it be all the holiday treats added to the stress of the season? Eating too much sugar doesn't just spike up your blood sugar or pack on the pounds. A study published in the *American Journal of Clinical Nutrition* found that eating one hundred grams of sugar (about one Big Gulp Coke) inhibited white blood cells from killing bacteria for up to five hours afterward.[2]

This study showed a 50 percent drop in the white blood cells' ability to engulf bacteria with the consumption of simple sugars like glucose, refined sugar, fructose, and honey. In contrast, consuming a complex carbohydrate (starch) solution did not affect the white blood cells' ability to engulf bacteria. Immune suppression was the highest two hours after consuming simple sugars, but after five hours the effects could still be seen.[3] People tend to overdose on sweets and beverages like sodas containing caffeine and sugar when studying, bored, or under stress. Stress alone will suppress the immune system, but when you add sugar, you have a double whopper. So people who consume sugary foods or beverages in order to cope with stress are actually weakening their health at the very time they need it in order to handle the stressful things that are going on.

If you get the flu or a cold, do you usually reach for a glass of orange juice? This is not the best choice, because orange juice is very high in sugar. It's interesting to note that sugar and vitamin C have a similar chemical structure. Sugar will actually compete with vitamin C for uptake into your immune cells. This means that the more sugar you eat, the less vitamin C you will be able to take into your white blood cells. And your white cells need plenty of vitamin C to stay strong. Sweets of all kinds will weaken your immune defense from infections.

A variety of other possibilities can weaken your immune system, which include physical and emotional stressors. There may be a possibility of a secondary bacterial infection to accompany a cold. Parasites and fungi can also harm the immune system. Even UV light can suppress the immune system, which can result in a greater susceptibility to cancer. And nutritional deficiencies and an unhealthy gut can also hinder immune function.

Healthy Gut, Healthy Immune System

The gut is responsible for 70 to 80 percent of the immune system function. Our intestinal flora influences this system. The gut mucosa communicates with the gastrointestinal immune cells, which come from the lymphoid branch of the immune system. Without ample good bacteria in the gut, the immune system can't do its job. Friendly bacteria are valuable. These little guys are mighty warriors. They enhance the "natural killer" effectiveness of immune cells and boost defenses to prevent pathogens and infectious agents from being absorbed.

Our gut flora is compromised when there's an overgrowth of unhealthy gut bacteria such as parasites and yeast like *Candida albicans*. The relationship between our gut flora and our immune systems is complex. For example, if you eat too much sugar, that can feed the opportunistic bacteria and they may increase to an unhealthy percentage. Or you may get a serious upper respiratory infection and need to take antibiotics. This can kill both the friendly and unfriendly gut bacteria and allow the opportunistic pathogens to get out of control. The hope is that we can bring balance to our gut flora. We want our "good bacteria" to live in harmony with the "unfriendly bacteria," and, most importantly, keep them in check.

When gut flora is at an optimal level, our digestion becomes more efficient and we reap the benefits from the production of short-chain fatty acids (SCFAs), which do many good things for us. SCFAs increase mitochondrial function (producing energy) and insulin sensitivity (allowing for a good blood sugar balance). Unfortunately this ideal condition is not a reality for many people. When friendly gut flora is disrupted or even lessened in number through antibiotic use, the consumption of too many sweets, or ongoing, chronic stress, the bad bacteria may become opportunistic and "take over the land." This can lead to intestinal permeability, or "leaky gut syndrome," systemic inflammation, and insulin insensitivity.

Our gut flora is like the TSA screening at the airport or security at a concert. It is there to keep undigested food, toxins, and pathogens from permeating the intestinal wall boundaries. When some of these things do get through, the good bacteria will signal the immune system to take action right away. It's like your home security alarm sounding off. Your gut flora signals the body of an intruder. If this happens frequently, the immune system must work overtime to capture the "bad guys" and snuff out the fires. This can overwhelm it so that it will stop functioning effectively.

Ten Tips to Enhance Your Immune System

1. **Avoid sugar.** Keep even healthy sweets to a minimum. Sugar undermines the health of white blood cells. It's important to minimize even natural sweeteners like honey and pure maple syrup. Avoid all artificial sweeteners. Even watch getting too much coconut nectar or stevia.

2. **Clean up your diet.** This is important so you will know what foods affect you. Go grain-free, dairy-free, and sugar-free.

3. **Take fish oil.** This helps to quell inflammation.

4. **Include a good probiotic.** A good probiotic in your diet, such as HMF Forte or Bio-Kult. Ingestible

probiotics are live microbial food supplements that can improve your intestinal flora. Though you may not need them every day, be sure to take them during stressful times, after antibiotics, when you travel, and when you get sick.

5. **Get plenty of sleep.** It's imperative to give your body ample downtime so that you can reset, reboot, and recharge. There is a large percentage of people in America who only get five or six hours of sleep a night. That is not enough! Most people need between seven hours and nine hours of sleep per night in a darkened room without interruptions. It's during the deep sleep that powerful healing hormones are released and your immune system is recharged.

6. **Ditch unhealthy fats.** Hunt down all polyunsaturated fats (vegetable oils such as corn, soy, safflower, and sunflower). Avoid canola; rapeseed is a big GMO product. These oils oxidize easily and adversely affect the immune system.

7. **Lose weight.** Carrying too much weight is not good for your immune system. Studies show that overweight people have less ability to fight off infection.

8. **Drink eight glasses of purified water each day.** This is a boost for the immune system and helps flush away toxins. Drink a glass of water first thing in the morning to cleanse your system.

9. **Exercise.** It has been proven to boost the immune system. Pick something you enjoy doing so you'll keep doing it.

10. **De-stress, meditate, pray, and relax.** Stress is called the silent killer. My husband, who is a psychotherapist, says it's the biggest problem we face today. We know that high levels of stress lead to a depressed immune system.

Supplements for Your Immune System

Because the immune system needs a lot of support, any decline in essential nutrients can have an adverse effect on our bodies. When nutrients are deficient, the body will use them for the brain, heart, and other vital organs, leaving less available for the immune system. To keep the immune system strong, we need plenty of these powerful nutrient helpers. We especially need nutrients with antioxidant capacity like vitamins C and E, selenium, beta-carotene, and other phytonutrients.

- Zinc is a trace mineral that is important for white blood cell function. Zinc deficiency affects the ability of T cells and other immune cells to function as they should. It has been shown in studies to zap a cold by shortening its duration if used within twenty-four hours of onset. Juice up zinc-rich foods such as ginger root, carrots, parsley, and garlic for a concentration of this powerhouse mineral.

- Vitamin A and carotenes play a central role in the development of immune cells. Many carotenes, including beta-carotene, are converted to vitamin A in the body as needed. Best juice sources include carrots, kale, parsley, spinach, beet greens, watercress, mangos, bell peppers, cantaloupe, and apricots.

- Vitamin B complex is especially important for proper immune functioning. Generally, the B vitamins are found in whole grains, liver, red meat, poultry, fish, eggs, nuts, and beans. The main juice source is green leafy vegetables.

- Vitamin C increases the health of white blood cells and antibodies. It also bumps up levels of interferon, which is the antibody that coats cell surfaces. This is very important to prevent the entrance of viruses. Best juice sources include bell peppers, kale, parsley, broccoli, brussels sprouts, cauliflower, cabbage, straw-berries, papayas, spinach, citrus fruits, mangos, and cantaloupe.

- Vitamin D was once known just for supporting strong bones. Now there is mounting evidence that it also affects the immune system. It has beneficial effects for the respiratory system. Vitamin D is created naturally in the skin through UV light. Supplemental vitamin D is necessary for many people who are deficient in this nutrient. Best food sources include egg yolk, sunflower seeds, tuna, sardines, beef, and cod liver oil.

- Folic acid is necessary to produce white blood cells (WBCs). In fact, taking too much folic acid increases WBCs. A deficiency of folic acid can cause anemia (low red blood cells). If you have low WBCs or are anemic, increasing folic acid may help. The best food sources include spinach, beans, and citrus fruits.

- Selenium is a trace mineral that has been shown in studies to help inflammation and immune responses. Selenium boosts the immune system and has been supported by studies involving aging, immunity, and protection against certain pathogens. Best food sources include lean meats, poultry, chicken, fish, seafood, beans, peas, eggs, nuts (especially Brazil nuts), and seeds.

- Coenzyme Q10 can be made by the body, but we may need more than the body can make at times of immuno- logical stress. Coenzyme Q10 (CoQ10) has a number of immune-enhancing effects, including increasing phagocytic activity and proliferation of granulocytes. Immune decline may be reversed with CoQ10 supple- mentation. Best food/juice sources include beef heart, sardines, peanuts, and spinach. CoQ10 supplements can be found at health food stores.

- Glutathione is an antioxidant important to lympho- cyte reproduction and T cell function. It is essential in recycling oxidized vitamins E and C. Best juice and food sources are asparagus, watermelon, citrus fruits, strawberries, peaches, cauliflower, broccoli, and tomatoes.

- Echinacea helps stimulate the immune system by increasing white blood cell production.

- Oleander extract is an herbal folk remedy for building up the immune system.

- Astragalus root can help stimulate white blood cells and also protect against invading organisms. It also promotes the production of interferon, which fights viruses.

- Green tea stimulates production of white blood cells.

- Garlic helps white blood cells fight infections and stimulates other immune cells. Rats that were fed garlic showed a significant increase in total white blood cell count.[4] Garlic is also known as a natural antibiotic.

Immune Symptom Dietary Recommendations

1. Eat a high-fiber, healthy fat diet.

2. Avoid sugar and alcohol. Studies have shown that consuming simple carbohydrates such as glucose, fructose, sucrose, honey, and orange juice all significantly reduced the ability of neutrophils to engulf and destroy bacteria.[5] (Alcohol is a simple carbohydrate.) Because of the high concentration of fruit sugar in fruit juice, limit your intake to no more than 4 ounces per day. Also, it is best to dilute fruit juice by half with water or a vegetable juice with a high water content, such as cucumber.

3. Eat more of your vegetables and fruits raw. Complex carbohydrates should make up the largest portion of your food choices, and of that group, raw vegetables and fruits should compose from 50 to 75 percent of this category. Raw foods are powerful caretakers of the immune system, offering vitamins, minerals, enzymes, essential oils, natural antibiotics, plant hormones, phytonutrients, and various forms of fiber. These raw foods are "alive" with the energy directly derived from the sun during photosynthesis. When we eat the plants, this special energy is passed to our body and thus our immune cells. That's where fresh vegetable juices and green smoothies can make it easy to consume more raw produce.

4. Drink fresh juice. Fresh juice equals pure immune power. Juices provide most of the benefits for the immune system that raw foods do, but with minimum strain on the digestive system. It is estimated that the nutrients are at work in the bloodstream within minutes of drinking them. Some juices have particular immune-enhancing qualities. Wheatgrass juice has been studied for its ability to inhibit mutations in DNA, garlic has antibiotic properties, and ginger is an anti-inflammatory. Cabbage juice is used for its anti-inflammatory, anti-ulcer, and antibiotic qualities.

5. Boost your immune system with a juice fast. Periodic juice fasting for one to three days is terrific for getting rid of toxins and waste. It helps the body eliminate poisons at the cellular level, gives the digestive

system a rest, and speeds up the white blood cells' ability to destroy diseased, damaged, and dead cells, along with giving the immune system a power boost. If you are not feeling your best, vegetable juice fasting for twenty-four to forty-eight hours can greatly benefit your immune system and get you back on your feet quickly.

Speed Up Healing!

Should you feed a cold and starve a fever? Yes and no. To speed your recovery, remember to eat light and drink nutrient-rich juices and smoothies along with plenty of water, herbal tea, and broth. This can make a big difference in your immune system response. When you eat light or spend a day vegetable juice fasting, you give your digestive system a rest from many hours of energy going toward digestion so it can concentrate on healing and repair work. On a normal day when you eat three meals, your body spends most of the day digesting what you ate. This does not allow much time for repair of the body. When you're sick, you need to feed your immune system a power pack of nutrients so it will have the antioxidants needed to outperform the bug. This is where fresh juice and green smoothies come to the rescue. They are packed with nutrients, broken down so they are easily digested, and put very little stress or strain on the digestive system. When you're under the weather, drink your way to a speedy recovery.

Whether a cold, the flu, bronchitis, or any other illness has taken you down, your food and beverage choices can make a huge difference as to whether you recover quickly or get worse and prolong your illness. You'll want to consume foods that dial down inflammation rather than fuel the fire. Cold symptoms such as mucus production and a runny nose are your body's inflammatory response to the pathogen.

Immune Building Recommendations

- Hydrate your body well, because dehydration causes much of the discomfort that is associated with a fever. Fluids also help to loosen and remove mucus from the body. Hot liquids help soothe a sore throat. Drink plenty of water and other fluids such as hot herbal tea—preferably two quarts of water per day to help you stay hydrated. Vegetable juices are also very helpful.

- Don't eat *any* sweets. Sugar can adversely impact your immune system and hinder its work.

- Alcohol and caffeine are very dehydrating; avoid them.

- Herbal tea is helpful, especially ginger and echinacea. Ginger root is a proven anti-inflammatory.

- Drink juices like greens with lemon and ginger, which reduce inflammation.

Include These Supplements

- Cysteine, an amino acid, helps thin mucus in the lungs and calms a cough and stuffy nose. Chicken is a good source of cysteine, so don't forget Grandma's chicken soup. She may not have known the science behind it, but she knew it helped. A 2000 study from the University of Nebraska Medical Center shows that chicken soup has anti-inflammatory properties that can soothe sore throats and bring relief for colds and flu.[6] Add lots of garlic for a natural antibiotic booster. Plus, the hot broth prevents dehydration and can comfort a sore throat.

- Beta-carotene is an antioxidant that supports immune function and mucous membrane health. The Institute of Food Research in the UK conducted a study in 1997 that suggests eating foods rich in beta-carotene enhances cell-mediated immune responses.[7] Include foods rich in carotenes such as carrots, collard greens, kale, parsley, spinach, chard, bell peppers, cantaloupe, apricots, broccoli, and romaine lettuce.

Healing Recipes

Anti-Inflammatory Cocktail

1 green apple
½ large fennel
1-inch piece ginger root
1 large broccoli stem
3 leaves kale
½ cucumber, peeled if not organic

Cut produce to fit your juicer. Start by juicing the apple and finish with the cucumber. Drink as soon as possible. Serves 2.

Notes: There are several benefits to each of these ingredients.
Fennel: anti-inflammatory, antihistamine, and antioxidant rich
Apple: rich in histamine-lowering quercetin
Cucumber: rich in antioxidants that help to prevent the synthesis of the inflammatory compound prostaglandin
Broccoli: anticarcinogenic, potential histamine-lowering action
Ginger: anti-inflammatory

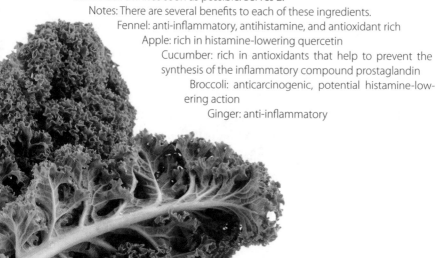

Cold and Flu Kicker Tonic[8]

32 oz. bottle organic apple cider vinegar
¼ cup chopped garlic
¼ cup chopped onions
¼ cup chopped hottest peppers available (or 1 small pepper)
¼ cup grated ginger
2 Tbsp. grated horseradish (or use premade if you can't find fresh)
2 Tbsp. turmeric

Blend and strain. Pour liquid back in the bottle. Discard the rest. Drink a 1-ounce shot a day.

Notes: Consume more garlic; it is considered a natural antibiotic.

Sore Throat Soother

Drink hot tea with lemon and honey. Black and green teas are rich in L-theanine—an antioxidant immune booster. Sip a cup or two and soothe a sore throat too.

Ginger Twister

From *The Juice Lady's Big Book of Juices and Green Smoothies*

You can give your immune system a "booster shot" with ginger—a powerful anti-inflammatory.

1 handful of parsley
1 kale leaf
1 apple
½ lemon, peeled if not organic
3 carrots, scrubbed well, tops removed, ends trimmed
2-inch chunk fresh ginger root

Cut produce to fit your juicer's feed tube. Wrap parsley in kale leaf and push slowly through juicer. Follow with remaining ingredients and stir. Pour into a glass and drink as soon as possible. Serves 1.

109

Make a Vitamin C-Rich Smoothie or Juice

Studies show that vitamin C can shorten the duration of a cold or flu. Produce rich in vitamin C includes bell peppers, kale, parsley, broccoli, citrus, strawberries, and cabbage. Pair these foods with foods rich in flavonoids. Studies suggest that flavonoids may support transport of vitamin C, a key immune-boosting nutrient that is needed to make disease-fighting antibodies. Flavonoids are known as antioxidants and are anti-inflammatory. Foods rich in flavonoids include citrus, parsley, cabbage, bell peppers, blackberries, and grapefruit.

Green Power Pro Smoothie

From *The Juice Lady's Big Book of Juices and Green Smoothies*

3 kale leaves, chopped
3 chard leaves, chopped
3 red leaf lettuce leaves, chopped
½ cup parsley, chopped
1 pear, stems removed, cut into chunks
½ banana, peeled, cut into chunks
½ cup almond or coconut milk

Combine all ingredients in a blender and process until smooth and creamy. Pour into glasses and serve immediately. Serves 2.

You Are Loved Cocktail

From *The Juice Lady's Anti-Inflammation Diet*

3 carrots, scrubbed well, tops removed, ends trimmed
2 ribs of celery with leaves
1 apple
1 cucumber, peeled if not organic
1 handful of spinach
1 lemon, peeled if not organic
½ beet, scrubbed well, with stems and leaves

Cut produce to fit your juicer's feed tube. Juice all ingredients and stir. Pour into a glass and drink as soon as possible. Serves 1–2.

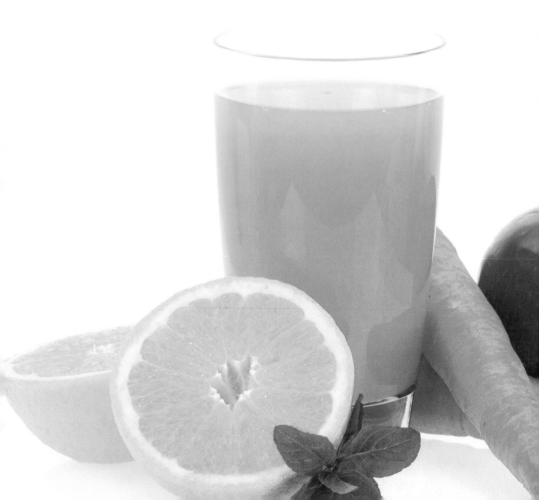

Chapter 7

SUCKER PUNCH THE EXTRA WEIGHT

HOW DOES SUGAR make you fat when it has no fat? Anytime you give your body more fuel than it needs, your liver's sugar storage tank (glycogen) fills up. Once the liver is full, any extra sugar is converted into fatty acids and travels through the bloodstream to be stored as fat in the places where the body tends to store fat. That could be the hips, stomach, thighs, buttocks, arms, or breasts. It spills over to your organs like the heart, liver, and kidneys, and compromises the ability to function well, raises blood pressure, decreases metabolism, and weakens the immune system. And that's just the beginning. In this chapter, we'll look at the many ways sugar causes the body to become fat and what we can do about it.

The Story of Excess Insulin

When we eat sweets, glucose levels go up. Glucose prompts the pancreas to secrete insulin. Insulin acts on cells in the liver, muscles, and fat tissues. It sends a command to the cells to go into action and do the following:

- Absorb glucose.
- Cease to break down glucose.
- Change glycogen into glucose.

- Produce glycogen from glucose.
- Make fats (triglycerides) from glycerol and fatty acids.
- Make proteins out of amino acids.

Insulin is released in excess anytime you ingest simple carbohydrates, which would include fruit juice, white bread, most wheat bread, white rice, white potatoes, muffins, bagels, jams, jelly, chips, croissants, pretzels, crackers, cookies, pancakes, breakfast cereal, cupcakes, sugary drinks, soft drinks, sports drinks, and beer—virtually all simple carbohydrates.[1]

When the body's fat-burning process stops, you stop burning glucose for energy. Then insulin will store sugar in muscles. When those energy stores are filled, the excess sugar will get converted to fat and stored in fat cells. Insulin promotes absorption of glycogen (blood glucose) in the liver. This can cause blood glucose to dip too low. That results in an increased appetite, and carb craving, which is then remedied by eating more carbs. At the same time, the body produces cortisol. Cortisol precipitates the release of stored sugar from the liver to return blood sugar levels to normal. If the body has difficulty accessing the stored sugar, the brain thinks it's hungry. Then you eat more, and the cycle spins on again. You gain weight and remain carb addicted.

Are Your Hormones Out of Whack?

The appetite-suppressing hormone in your body is called leptin, which is adversely affected by the consumption of sugar. Leptin is released by fat cells; the heftier those fat cells are, the more leptin will be secreted. The brain depends upon this signaling hormone to determine how much fat should be stored up for a rainy day. Therefore, the more sugar we eat, the more fat will be stored in our fat cells. And the more fat is stored, the more they balloon up, and the more leptin they secrete. Leptin sends a message to the brain that we've eaten enough. This is the marvelous mechanism we have been given to keep us from eating on and on and to prevent us from becoming obese. Increased leptin also prompts cells to release more fat and raises the metabolic rate. However, the whacky problem occurs when the body becomes resistant to leptin. This means that it doesn't recognize leptin in the blood. Then the regulation breaks down. This is called "leptin resistance." This imbalance makes us fat, because our checks and balances have broken down. Ghrelin, the appetite-stimulating hormone, shoots up, and the brain thinks we need food. It therefore prompts us to eat more and burn fewer calories. Try exerting your willpower over ghrelin-driven hunger signals! It's next to impossible.

So what causes leptin resistance in the first place? A high-sugar diet. Sugar raises triglycerides. This blocks the transport of leptin to the brain and throws body fat regulation out of whack. Then the brain signals that we need to keep eating. The urge can seem unstoppable.

This body-brain connection of food regulation is very complex. Think hormones and neurological circuits. The hypothalamus is where signals are interpreted, and it is ground zero where leptin is recognized, along with neurons and other hormones.

In 2013 one study considered the effects of fructose versus glucose on satiety (feelings of being full) and food consumption. The researchers fed twenty healthy volunteers either a glucose-sweetened drink or a fructose-sweetened drink. The brains of the volunteers were scanned, and then they were asked various questions. The glucose drink seemed to lower activity and blood flow in the hypothalamus, but the fructose drink did not. The glucose drinkers weren't as hungry and they felt more satiated compared to the fructose drinkers, who reported they didn't feel satisfied at all; they were still hungry after the drink. The conclusion of the researchers was that the fructose drink did not produce satiety.[2]

A different study showed that fructose did not, in fact, reduce ghrelin (the body's appetite-stimulating hormone) the way that glucose did. The more ghrelin the body produces, the more we want to eat. In order to eat less, we must reverse leptin resistance, so that the brain will get the message that we've had enough to eat.

Is it a high-sugar and high-carbs diet or a high-fat one that is driving America's obesity epidemic? *Why We Get Fat* author Gary Taubes explains that carbs, including fructose, can destroy insulin and leptin sensitivity. This causes cells to collect more fat, making it difficult to lose extra weight.[3]

It's an Acid Problem

You just downed a sports drink and a "slimming" energy bar. It seemed like a good choice after your workout, right? It's not. When we look at this combo regarding weight loss and alkaline-acid balance, it's a poor choice. Sports drinks can be among the most acidic things we can drink. In fact, these drinks are so acidic that they promote tooth erosion. One dentist in Great Britain looked at the acidity of eight different sports drinks after examining a twenty-three-year-old runner who had severely eroded front teeth. The runner had often quenched his thirst with sports drinks. All eight drinks analyzed were below the normal safe pH of 5.5.[4]

As for the popular energy bars—they all contain some sweetener, even the "thin" ones. Check the label. The thin ones I looked at had maltitol—a sugar alcohol. Sweeteners are acidic. They also set you up for a glycemic response and ultimately insulin resistance.

This is just one example of typical American choices that are either acidic or turn acidic when digested, thus creating mild acidosis, weight gain, and ill health.

Your body must maintain a delicate, precise pH balance in the blood, which is slightly alkaline. A healthy pH blood balance should be between 7.35 and 7.45. To maintain this balance the body will even draw minerals from bones, teeth, and muscles if it must to use as a buffer against the acids.

The acidity or alkalinity of foods can be classified by how we process them. Our bodies transform nearly all foods into acid or alkaline bases. Though we need a balance of different foods for good health, most people eat far more acid-producing foods than alkaline-forming foods. Consuming too many acid-forming substances causes a chronic condition known as acidosis, which means the body has become too acidic. Additionally, acid is produced in your body whenever you experience stress or strong emotions. You can see that the typical Western diet and lifestyle moves us in the wrong direction. Dr. Robert Young, author of *The pH Miracle*, has been saying for years that obesity is an acid problem and that fat is saving our lives because our bodies will store acid in fat cells to protect our vital organs and tissues.

Are You Overacidic?

What happens to your body when you're overly acidic? Acids act on your tissues like meat tenderizer on a New York strip. Acid cooks your organs and tissues. Look no further than ceviche (fresh raw seafood cooked in citrus juices). The body will do whatever it can to protect your precious organs from this caustic action. What can't be neutralized is most often stored in fat cells to protect vital and more delicate parts. The body will even make more fat cells for storage as needed. That means we could gain more and more weight while not even overeating—just by eating the wrong foods.

This slightly acidic condition also sets us up for weak bones and teeth. Over time, the body will leach calcium from bones and teeth to act as buffers to neutralize acids and maintain the pH balance in the blood. This could account for one reason why osteoporosis is on the rise.

Overacidity also contributes to the deterioration of muscles, since magnesium is leached out of muscles to act as a buffer for the acid. Could this account for one reason we're seeing a drastic increase in fibromyalgia—a condition characterized by muscle and joint pain that is often helped by magnesium supplementation? This is why I encourage juicing magnesium-rich vegetables such as chard, collards, spinach, beet tops, and other hearty greens.

If all of that is not enough to get your attention, too much acid also contributes to inflammation (a major factor in heart disease), aging (including the skin), and kidney stones. If you want to look younger and prevent diseases caused by inflammation, it's very wise to eat an alkaline-rich diet, as presented in the recipes and menu plan in my book *The Juice Lady's Turbo Diet*.

Alkaline Balance Contributes to a Strong Metabolism

The blood plays a very important role in your health—it carries oxygen and nutrients to all the cells. When your blood is optimally pH balanced, it carries oxygen more efficiently. Oxygen contributes to a strong metabolism, gives you energy, and keeps you healthy. It also plays a key role in how well you sleep. Blood cells tend to clump together in a more acidic environment. Healthy red blood cells are spaced apart from each other. Consequently the blood can move freely throughout the body, and it even gets into the small capillaries. As a result, you may feel like your whole body is energized.

During deep sleep, proper blood flow is important for healing and repair. When your blood is healthy, your sleep is energizing and rejuvenating and you need less of it. Conversely research confirms that when we don't sleep well, we tend to eat more food, especially the fattening, high-carb (acidic) kinds that pack on the pounds. Also, without ample oxygen, our metabolism slows down, and food digests more slowly, causing weight gain, sluggishness, and food fermentation, which contributes to yeast overgrowth, fungus, and mold throughout the body. These pathogens can cause weight gain and an inability to lose weight.

Why Veggie Juices Facilitate Weight Loss

One important factor when juicing vegetables and drinking green smoothies is alkalinity. Achieving a 75 percent alkaline to a 25 percent acid balance in foods and beverages and regulating your body's acid/alkaline chemistry through simple dietary changes can result in weight loss, increased energy, and a greater sense of well-being.

Throughout history until the last century, most people's diets were more alkaline than acidic. Because most people couldn't catch or afford a lot of meat, they relied more on vegan foods such as beans, whole grains, and vegetables. Today, people rely heavily on animal products as the main part of their diet. Research shows that eating lots of animal protein produces excess acid, but a diet dominant in plant foods promotes a slightly alkaline pH-balanced system. A German study of 720 children revealed that those who ate more fruits and vegetables produced less acid than those eating more meat, dairy, eggs, and grains. Acidic foods and beverages include meat, poultry, eggs, dairy, fish, oxidized oils, trans fats, sweets, soda, sports drinks, coffee, black tea, alcohol, junk food, and many grains.

Once you stop ingesting a large quantity of acidic foods and beverages, the body doesn't have to hang on to fat cells as it did before. As the acid/alkaline balance becomes healthier, the body can then haul off a bunch of those little fat storage units. You can celebrate! Your metabolism will perk up because your adrenal and thyroid function will improve. Listen up! That happens because too much acid impairs thyroid and adrenal function, meaning there will be a drop in the hormones needed for a fired-up metabolism. With slow hormone activity, the body won't turn fat and calories into energy as easily. Many people in this condition say they don't eat a lot of food and should be losing weight, but they just can't seem to drop even a pound or two when they're very strict.

I've looked at many dieters' diaries, and have found that often people are indeed eating small portions and still not losing weight. Alas, in those cases, it's what they're eating rather than the quantity. With an alkalizing, nutrient-rich diet that helps to get your hormones back in balance, enzyme production and metabolism get "up and going!"

Adding high-alkaline vegetable juices to your diet makes weight loss easier than ever, because not only are the juices alkaline, they are already broken down and simple to digest. That means they are used quickly to alkalize and energize your body. And they are packed with minerals and other nutrients that help you achieve an acid-alkaline balance without leaching minerals from your bones, teeth, and muscles. And that spells better health in the future as well as a trimmer body.

NITA LOST FORTY-TWO POUNDS

In early July 2008 I read the best article on detoxing I have ever read in the *PCC Sound Consumer* (a newsletter from the Seattle area PCC markets) written by Cherie Calbom. Having gone through a recent divorce and a weight gain of fifty pounds over the past year and a half, I really needed to cleanse physically, emotionally, and spiritually. I immediately went to the bookstore and purchased her book *Juicing, Fasting, and Detoxing for Life*. I began by eating only foods from the alkaline food list, and avoiding most foods from the acidic list. I also increased my water intake. By the end of July I had lost eight pounds just doing this alone. I then began juicing. I also tried a nine-day juice cleanse. I dropped another twelve pounds—totaling twenty pounds in the first month! I ate all organic whole foods, and about 90 percent of that was raw. My energy level increased dramatically, enabling me to start jogging—actually it was more like "chugging." Then I started Cherie's colon cleanse program, and subsequently lost another twenty pounds.

I lost a total of 42 pounds in a mere twelve weeks into my new lifestyle. I started at 168 pounds. I now weigh 126. I'll also be trying Cherie's liver-gallbladder cleanse and her kidney cleanse.

I'm an aesthetician and have influenced several of my clients and colleagues at the hotel spa where I work. Many of them have purchased Cherie's books and are enjoying wonderful results of their own. I feel so good about starting this juicing and healthy lifestyle movement at our downtown spa.

(You can view Nita's before and after pictures at http://www.juiceladycherie.com/Juice/success-stories/.)

—Nita

What Is pH?

The pH range is from 0 to 14, with 7.0 being neutral. Anything above 7.0 is alkaline; anything below 7.0 is considered acidic. The pH is the measurement of the acidity or alkalinity of a solution, which is the actual measurement of hydrogen ions. The letters *pH* stand for the potential of hydrogen; "H" is capitalized because it's the symbol for hydrogen. An increase in hydrogen ions (less bonding) results in a drop of the pH (more acidic), while a decrease in hydrogen ions results in a pH rise (more alkaline). The higher the pH reading, the more alkaline the solution. The lower the pH reading, the more acidic the solution.

As I mentioned earlier, human blood pH should be slightly alkaline, between 7.35 and 7.45. The body continually strives to keep this balance. When it's compromised, many problems can occur. Just a slight pH imbalance can bring about feelings of fatigue, cause weight gain, promote trouble with food digestion, and cause many different aches and pains. Most parts of the body have different ranges of pH. The skin can vary from 4.5 to 7.0, and stomach acid can range from 1.0 to 3.0. Pancreatic secretions themselves may range from 8.0 to 8.3. However, the blood range must be very narrow. If the pH of your blood gets even slightly outside of this very narrow range, you can become sick. If it deviates too far from the acceptable range for very long, you could go into shock, fall into a coma, or even die. Severe acidosis such as this is rare, but mild acidosis is becoming much more common, and it is thought to affect at least half of the population.

How to Test Your pH

By analyzing your body's fluids, you can measure what's going on inside your body. It's a good practice to either test one hour before or two hours after eating. You can test your urine and saliva with litmus test strips that you can typically find at drugstores.

Saliva pH Test

When you test your saliva, fill your mouth with saliva and then swallow. This helps remove acidic bacteria. Don't rinse your mouth before testing the saliva because this will record the alkalinity of the water or other liquid you used. Wet a piece of litmus paper with your saliva. While generally more acidic than blood, salivary pH mirrors the blood. It is a fair indicator of the extracellular fluids of your body. Saliva pH levels can range anywhere from 5.5 to 7.5 or more. The optimal pH for saliva is 6.5 to 7.5. A reading lower than 6.5 indicates an insufficient reserve of alkaline. After you eat, your saliva pH should rise to 7.5 or above. If there are enough minerals in your system, your saliva test should register from 7.0 to 7.5. But if your mineral reserves are too low, you will typically test at a 6.4 or below. Some people test as low as 4.5 to 5.75. (Keep in mind that the pH scale works like the Richter scale; it's logarithmic. A pH of 5.0 is 100 times too acidic.) If your pH tests are that low (acidic), you should take immediate action to correct the problem by increasing your minerals and drinking vegetable juices that are rich in dark leafy greens and green stalks such as broccoli, asparagus stems, and broccoli stems mixed with cucumber, carrot, and lemon (very alkaline).

Urine pH Test

When testing your urine, let some urine flow before catching it. This will give a more accurate reading. The pH of the urine indicates how the body is working to maintain the proper pH of the blood. The pH of urine points out the efforts of the body to regulate pH through the buffer system. Urine can provide a fairly accurate picture of body chemistry, since values are based on your body's elimination. Urine pH can vary from 4.5 to 9.0, but the ideal range should be 6.0 to 7.0. Urinary pH can fluctuate from 6.0 to 6.5 first thing in the morning and between 6.5 and 7.0 in the evening before you eat dinner. This would be the healthy range.

A urine test can indicate how efficient your body is in excreting acids and assimilating the minerals you need, particularly calcium, magnesium, sodium, and potassium. These minerals function as buffers, substances that help balance the body and protect it from too much acidity or too much alkalinity. If your buffering system becomes overwhelmed, you should immediately work to restore it through diet and stress reduction.

A big difference can exist between your urine and saliva readings because your mouth is naturally more acidic. If you brush your teeth, the reading will show a higher alkaline reading due to the toothpaste and water. Your urine will usually reflect your body's process of removing acid.

A person who eats a typical American diet is more likely to have a saliva pH average between 5.5 and 6.0. At first this may not seem much lower than the normal range, but this is based on a logarithmic scale—in which each step is ten times the previous step. For example, 5.5 is 100 times more acidic than 6.5.

If you test your saliva or urine pH, you will then have an idea of the general trend your body is taking. Unfortunately, however, there is no way of determining the exact pH of your blood without undergoing a live blood analysis.

How the Acid-Alkaline Value of Food Is Determined

Acid-alkaline diet food chart quantifications come from the pH of the ash that results from the body burning food for fuel. The alkaline/acid value is determined by measuring unused minerals. Digestion produces an ash, a residue that is still left after we digest foods. It's this ash that can be measured to determine whether the foods are alkaline or acid. When we digest a certain food, it is chemically oxidized; in other words, it is burned to form water, carbon dioxide, and an inorganic compound. The inorganic compound determines whether the food is alkaline or acid producing. If it contains more sodium, potassium, or calcium, it's considered an alkaline food. If it contains more sulfur, phosphate, or chloride, it's classified as an acidic food.

The Alkaline and Acid Foods

Inconsistencies among the various lists exist, and so I go by a general guideline to consider: meat, dairy, grains, sugar, coffee, tea, alcohol, junk food, soda pop, and fast food are considered acidic in their final breakdowns, and vegetables, fruit, sprouts, seeds, nuts, and legumes are considered alkaline. Some practitioners go by their own personal experience when dealing with clients, along with measurements with litmus paper and health results achieved by reducing the acid-forming foods. I've had good results in working with people to help them reduce the acid-forming foods they eat and consuming more alkaline-forming foods.

Regardless of research or lack thereof, the principles are clear: consume plenty of vegetable juices, green smoothies, vegetables, sprouts, fruit, nuts, and seeds, and eat sparingly dairy products, grains, and protein from eggs, meat, and fish. You don't have to cut out all acid-forming foods; about 25 percent of our diet should be from acid-forming foods and the rest from alkaline-forming foods. This may mean that you need to shift the overall balance of your diet toward vegan foods (the alkaline group) and away from excessively eating the acid-forming foods, which is typically the diet of a fast-food culture. Don't worry if there are days here and there when your day looks more like a fifty/fifty split or leans even more toward the acid-forming foods. It's what you do on most days that matters.

Most health professionals agree that this list is fairly accurate when it comes to acid- and alkaline-forming foods.

Acidic Foods	Alkaline Foods
Meat	Vegetable juices
Poultry	Vegetables
Eggs	Sprouts
Dairy	Fruit
Fish	Seeds and nuts
Grains	Legumes (beans, lentils, split peas)
Trans fats	
Sugar and sweets	
Soda	
Sports drinks	
Coffee	
Black tea	
Alcohol (wine, beer, liquor)	
Junk food	

DR. HAY'S EXPERIMENT

Dr. Howard Hay developed high blood pressure, Bright's disease (kidney disease), and a dilated heart in 1908 after he had practiced medicine for sixteen years. He could find no treatment for his problems available, so he decided to search for a cure himself. His investigation led him to the chemistry of digestion, the essential enzymes involved in the process, and foods' acidifying or alkalizing effects on the body. After he changed his diet, his colleagues were amazed by the complete remission of his symptoms and diseases in just three months. He also lost about forty-five pounds. In 1911 he introduced his program, which entailed food-combining guidelines, where he emphasized proper food combining and the reduction of acid-forming foods.[5]

Science in Support of an Alkaline Diet

Starting around age forty-five, we begin to lose some of our alkaline buffer bicarbonates (minerals). One study at the University of California showed that dominant acid-forming diets produce a low-grade systemic metabolic acidosis in healthy adults. As we age, the degree of acidosis increases.[6]

The *American Journal of Clinical Nutrition* concluded that alkalizing diets improve bone density and growth hormone concentrations, whereas acidic diets contribute to bone and muscle loss. In one study at the University of Chicago, "participants consumed a low carbohydrate, high protein diet for six weeks. They all produced more acid in their urine and showed signs of increased risk of kidney stone formation and bone loss."[7]

In his book *Reverse Aging* Sang Whang says that we age because we accumulate acidic wastes over time. The wastes include uric acid, urate, sulfate, phosphate, kidney stones, and organic wastes often surrounded by cholesterol. Cellulite is made up of fat, toxins, and water in which toxins and acidic wastes are trapped in cottage cheese–looking pockets below the skin.[8]

Are Toxins Making You Fat and Sick?

In 2008 scientists discovered this surprising fact: "Environmental toxins make you fat and cause diabetes."[9] Chemicals disturb the body's ability to balance blood sugar and metabolize cholesterol.

These disruptions can promote insulin resistance. Why hasn't this been headline news? Probably because there are no drugs to treat it. In fact, the drugs would only add to the toxicity. In our efforts to conquer diabetes and obesity, two of the biggest epidemics we face today, we must look at the environmental toxins, food toxins, cleaning products, and beauty products that we use on our bodies.

It is imperative that you optimize your body's ability to detox. If your detoxification tools aren't up to speed, waste will build up in your organs and tissues. This toxic buildup is similar to what happens when trash collectors go on strike. Waste piles up high, creating bad smells and a breeding ground for illness. Do you remember the New York City Christmas Trash Collectors Strike of 1981? Trash mounded up in the streets, which attracted rats in droves and led to disease. Had it not been so cold, they would have had a major health crisis. When the trash was finally hauled away, with nothing left to feed on, the rats left. Just like hauling away city trash, there is less for parasites, yeast, and fungus to feed on when we get rid of toxins.

Our environment is marinated in chemicals that our bodies were not designed to handle. The Centers for Disease Control and Prevention's National Report on Human Exposure to Environmental Chemicals gives an alarming look at the chemicals that invade our bodies. Scientists found that nearly every person tested was packing a plethora of nasty chemicals, which included "flame retardants stored in fatty tissue and Bisphenol A (BPA), a hormone-like substance found in plastics."[10] Even little babies were contaminated. "The average newborn has 287 chemicals in her umbilical cord blood, 217 of which are neurotoxic (poisonous to nerves or nerve cells)."[11]

And just as with acid, the body will store toxins in fat cells and not let go unless there are plenty of antioxidants to bind them and carry them away harmlessly. Toxins are big contributors to weight gain because your body will even make more fat cells in which to store toxins if it runs out of storage space. That is why an antioxidant-rich diet and vegetable juices in particular are so important to weight loss. It's also why a sugar-free diet is imperative. Sugar is toxic. You've read the studies I've reported. Sugar contributes to weight gain in so many ways, and one is its high toxicity. Sugar offers a medium for pathogens to grow. Get rid of your body's toxic waste, and just like New York City's rats left when the trash was hauled away, many physical problems will disappear.

HOLLY LOST THREE HUNDRED POUNDS GIVING UP SUGAR

I am here to tell you that it is not what I eat that has contributed to my weight loss so much as what I do NOT eat. And what I do NOT eat anymore is sugar. If there was any possible way that I could adequately convey to you the very real dangers of sugar, I would do it. If I could write in all caps or send warning sounds through this screen, I still could not adequately convey to you just how critical getting off sugar has been in my life. In 2003 I went on a low-carb diet and for the first time truly experienced a relief from cravings. I learned that cutting out sugar and carefully monitoring other food sources that gave me trouble was a key to keeping myself from feeling constantly hungry. This was a light bulb moment for me, and I lost 104 pounds by avoiding these trigger foods. Then I gained it all back plus more. Until I was over 400 pounds.

And now the pain. The excruciating, backbreaking pain. Swollen feet. Almost unable to walk. Unable to fit in most any chair. Almost unable to even fit behind the steering wheel of the car.

My life was about pain. Emotional and physical pain. Now I'm losing three hundred pounds. One pound at a time. I have discovered a faith that sustains me and gives me strength far better than cupcakes. (You can read more about Holly's incredible story and see her pictures at http://www.300poundsdown .com/2013/06/sugar-addiction-detox-and-gaining-control-over-food.html.)[12]

—Holly

Losing the Weight Recap

1. Get off sugar completely; see chapter 9 for the plan.

2. Alkalize your body.

3. Cleanse your body; get the toxins out.

Curb It!

Jerusalem artichoke juice combined with carrot is a traditional remedy for satisfying cravings for sweets and junk food. The key is to sip it slowly when you get a craving for high-fat or high-carb foods.

3-4 carrots, scrubbed well, tops removed, ends trimmed
2 celery ribs
1 Jerusalem artichoke, scrubbed well
1 cucumber, peeled if not organic
1 lemon, peeled if not organic
½ green apple

Cut produce to fit your juicer's feed tube. Juice ingredients and stir. Pour into a glass and drink as soon as possible. Serves 1.

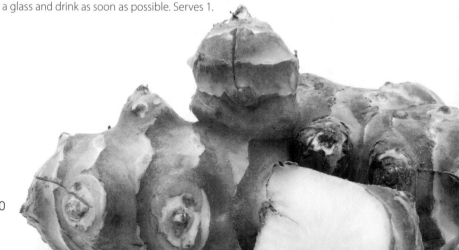

Chapter 8

THE SUGAR SHOPPING GUIDE

SUGAR IS THE general name for sweet, short-chain carbohydrates that are used in food preparation. Composed of carbon, hydrogen, and oxygen, they are simple sugars called monosaccharides and include glucose (dextrose, glucose produced from corn), fructose, ribose, xylose, and galactose. The primary sources of sugar that are commonly used in food preparation are sugarcane and sugar beets. These disaccharides are made up of one molecule of glucose bound to a molecule of sucrose.

Don't be fooled. This sweet stuff is hidden in packaging in so many different forms it could make your head spin: barley malt, beet sugar, brown sugar, buttered syrup, cane juice, cane juice crystals, cane juice solids, caramel, carob syrup, corn syrup, corn syrup solids, date sugar, dehydrated cane juice, dehydrated fruit juice, dextrin, diastase, diastatic malt, fruit juice, fruit juice concentrate, fruit juice crystals, golden syrup, high-fructose corn syrup, malt syrup, maltitol, maltodextrin, maple syrup, refiner's sugar, sorghum syrup, turbinado, and yellow sugar.

Are we being deceived about the amount of sugar that is in the products that we eat? The group at Food Matters says that we are. They note that "if a manufacturer wants to sweeten up a certain brand of crackers, it can either do this using 15 grams of 'sugar' or 5 grams of 'malt syrup,' 5 grams of 'invert sugar,' and 5 grams of 'glucose.'"[1] This makes the sugars appear low because they are noted in small amounts on the label of ingredients. This "divide-and-masquerade method" seems to be the route many manufacturers are going. The public believes the amount of sugar in the product they are buying is smaller than it is, but add it up and you may be shocked. Once you use this chapter as your shopping guide, you'll be outsmarting them.

Avoid the Bad Boys of the Sweet World

It is so important to limit the amount of sugar we eat, but in order to do that it is important to learn the many names for all of the "sweet stuff" that food manufacturers place on their labels. Sweeteners can come in so many different forms and go by so many different names that looking for it on a label can actually make you feel like a detective. Two clever ways that manufacturers have used to disguise sugar on food labels is through citing long, scientific words or even renaming the sugar altogether. It's past time to get acquainted with these names; begin to shop with a magnifying glass if you need to, because that is the other thing that manufacturers do—they make the print so small that no one can read it! But armed with a little knowledge, you'll quickly become an expert at spotting sweeteners on labels.

White Sugar (Table Sugar)

White refined sugar is sold as table sugar, baker's or bar sugar (superfine), sugar cubes, and powdered or confectioner's sugar. Do you remember that commercial jingle for sugar from way back down memory lane? Sounds so natural; looks so beautiful. But it's not so beautiful when it comes to the processing part.

Processing sugar involves separation of crystals from the liquid pulp of sugarcane or sugar beets, which produces molasses. (Be aware: 50 percent of white sugar sold in the United States is made from sugar beets, and 95 percent of the sugar beets are genetically modified.) Sugar has all the beneficial nutrients that were in the original plant—vitamins, minerals, enzymes, and phytonutrients—stripped away. But that's not all. Unless you purchase unbleached cane sugar, you will be consuming residues of the chemicals used in bleaching and refining. Look at sulfur dioxide, a type of sulfite. If you have asthma, sulfite sensitivity, or sulfite allergy, this can contribute to allergy-like symptoms. Also, the effects of sulfur dioxide on the environment are very detrimental. Acidifying compounds are formed when sulfur dioxide and nitrogen oxides are combined with water in the earth's atmosphere and then deposited on the earth. There, they can cause acidification of soil and lakes.

Phosphoric acid, used in processing sugar, is a clear, colorless, odorless, highly acidic liquid that has been linked to lower bone density in some epidemiological studies, including a study published in the *American Journal of Clinical Nutrition*.[2] Calcium hydroxide, which is slaked lime, is often used in sugar processing as well. The National Institutes of Health warns that it is toxic and can introduce serious health problems as a result of various types of exposure. In small residues it probably doesn't cause much damage, but what about buildup over time?

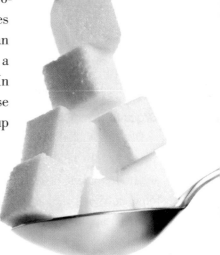

Wake up and smell the coffee... without a sugar cube. Commercial sweets such as cakes, cookies, candies, and ice cream usually contain white table sugar that has all the other detrimental residues included too.

Evaporated Cane Juice

Evaporated cane juice is used in thousands of products today and often shows up in health food products. But is it any healthier than plain white sugar? Not much, say the experts. It is less processed, so it retains some trace minerals and doesn't have the bleaching residues, but it has the same amount of calories, carbs, and fructose, and therefore, similar deleterious effects on the body as refined sugar.

It is made by crushing sugarcane in large roller mills. Sweet cane juice is forced out, and the fiber and dirt are removed. The juice is made into syrup by boiling off the water in a process called evaporation. The syrup is then transferred to large pans and boiled, which is the last stage of the process, where more water is boiled off until the juice crystallizes. Once the crystals start to form, the primary liquid is spun in centrifuges to separate the crystals from the liquid. Then the sugar crystals are given a final drying using hot air before they are ready for shipment.

This sugar is being sold to green consumers by touting the fact that less-refined sugar requires less fossil fuel to produce, and that the transportation chain and the refining process are shorter. This is better for the environment, but it's still sugar. It is not good for you.

Organic Raw Cane Sugar

Don't be fooled: organically grown cane sugar is just sugar. There are a lot of "health products" sweetened with raw, organic cane sugar. It makes little difference that it is raw, except it contains more nutrients and the damaging heat used for refined sugar has not been applied along with a host of chemicals for bleaching. Your body will still recognize it as sugar, however. It will break it down into glucose and fructose in the digestive tract, and it will have the exact same effects on your metabolism. This is the darling of the health food industry today. But there's little difference between raw and refined sugar in the end. This is why raw, organic cane sugar is on my "bad boy" list.

High-Fructose Corn Syrup

For a long time, high-fructose corn syrup (HFCS) was the sweetener that was the most commonly consumed. HFCS is actually 55 percent fructose, and 45 percent of it is mostly glucose. This danger was first introduced to the market in the late 1970s and it seemed innocuous. Created to be indistinguishable from refined sugar, it was used primarily in soft drinks in the beginning.[3]

Though it is marketed as natural, HFCS is far from what grows in the sweet cornfields of Iowa where I grew up. Most sweet corn we eat off the cob is not genetically modified (GM), but white cornstarch and HFCS is mostly processed from genetically modified organisms (GMOs) and used to produce glucose, which is converted into fructose using high heat. A study by the Institute of Agriculture and Trade Policy (2009) revealed that some of the HFCS syrup is manufactured with "mercury-grade caustic soda."[4] This can cause mercury to accumulate in the body, which is especially damaging to the developing brain of a fetus as well as infants. This should be of particular concern for pregnant women. Overexposure to mercury can disrupt the development of our children.

HFCS adversely impacts the thyroid gland. Because it contains traces of mercury, it can disrupt thyroid function. Mercury is known as an endocrine disruptor. It competes for the same receptors in the thyroid gland that capture iodine. Iodine is essential for good thyroid health. Without this trace mineral, your thyroid gland is unable to produce thyroid hormones.

Because of the way HFCS is metabolized in the liver, it does not cause the pancreas to release insulin the way the body normally does. It is converted to fat more readily than any other sugars. Kidney specialists at the University of Florida discovered that fructose raised levels of uric acid in the blood, which then led to metabolic syndrome.[5] Harvard Health Publications has reported on studies that showed excess fructose caused fatty liver disease, making the liver look like that of an alcoholic.[6] The American Chemical Society warned that HFCS-sweetened soda contains high levels of reactive compounds that can trigger cell and tissue damage along with causing diabetes, particularly in children.[7]

Besides soda, HFCS has been used in breakfast cereals, stovetop stuffing, fruit drinks, frappuccinos, some breads and muffins, breakfast pastries, candy bars, ketchup, Miracle Whip, cookies, cakes, crackers, some dairy products, relish, pickles, ice cream, jams, jellies, syrups, salad dressings, sauces, lunch snacks, and some soups.

For a while the public viewed HFCS as a healthy alternative to "real" sugar. Manufacturers especially loved it because it was cheaper to use than sugar, so it was attractive for them to use widely in their products. However, we have now begun to see the real effects of what HFCS has done to our bodies, and refined sugar is making a comeback as the "healthful alternative" to corn syrup. Industry after industry is now replacing HFCS with sucrose and proudly advertising their products as having no high-fructose corn syrup. Unfortunately, however, both sweeteners still have similar biological effects, and plain old refined sugar is not such a lovely little switch.

Brown Sugar

Brown sugar is white sugar with small amounts of molasses added back in. When brown sugar is manufactured, bleached sugar is combined with sulfured molasses, which is molasses treated with sulfur dioxide as a preservative. Depending on the molasses added, various grades of brown sugar are produced—from light to dark. Some people claim that brown sugar is healthier than white. But regardless of the color, it's just plain old white sugar with a little molasses for coloring. Typical food products that contain brown sugar are bakery products, cereals, and baked goods.

Sucanat, Rapadura, and Turbinado Sugar

Rapadura and Sucanat are the brand names of dried sugarcane juice, and contrary to popular opinion they are not good for you. The process to produce Sucanat separates the sugar from the molasses, and then some molasses is added back in to give the final product a light golden color. The molasses is not removed at all in the process used to create Rapadura, which means that it ultimately has a darker color. It has more nutrients than the other two sugars.

Turbinado sugar is similar to Sucanat in that the molasses has been removed, but it has been more processed than Sucanat. Turbinado is almost exactly the same as table sugar, with the exception that it has not been bleached.

All three brands have the same level of sweetness as table sugar. They are typically advertised as healthy because they contain more nutrients, but there are only traces of nutrients present in these sugars. Most often, these forms of sugar are sold for home cooking. They are all sugar and react in the system with the same adverse effects.

Dextrose

Dextrose has been used by the American public for a long time; it's the old name for what we now call glucose. It is made up of equal parts of sucrose and fructose, usually produced from corn. An active form of glucose, dextrose has the same caloric value as table sugar; it is sweeter than sucrose but not as sweet as fructose. Unfortunately, dextrose is everywhere: It is added to a variety of foods such as cookies, ice cream, and sports drinks like Gatorade. It shows up in dehydrated green beans, fish sticks, and potato chips. It's also used in intravenous solutions in hospitals! Be aware that most dextrose that comes from corn has been genetically modified, because field corn is one of the biggest GMO crops in this country. The impact on our health and the environment from these crops is immense. It has a high glycemic index of 100. Unfortunately, dextrose shows up in a lot of products, and people don't even know what it is. Run from this sweetener; it's really bad.

Levulose

An older name for fructose, levulose is found in honey and ripened fruits. It is a combination of equal parts sucrose and glucose, and it has the same caloric value as refined sugar. It's sweeter than glucose and sucrose, but it is metabolized differently. It is purified for commercial sale by boiling inulin, a starch contained in dahlia tubers, with water; by the breakdown of cane sugar into glucose and fructose; or by reacting sucrose with sulfuric acid to achieve the breakdown. It is sweeter than cane sugar, and is more easily absorbed. Because it has a lower glycemic index than glucose or sucrose, it has been recommended for diabetics. But research indicates it actually has a negative impact on fat metabolism. I do not recommend it for diabetics—or anyone, for that matter. It bypasses the normal breakdown process and goes right to the liver, making it less desirable than other sweeteners. It's another sweetener to avoid completely.

Fructose

Fructose is the natural sugar found in fruit, honey, and some vegetables. Fructose is manufactured by treating corn with enzymes, which yields corn syrup. Manufactured fructose, which is cheap and used in many commercial products where you find corn sweetener, is sweeter than sugar, but it is digested much differently. Upon absorption fructose is sent directly to the liver, where it releases enzymes that actually tell the body to store fat. In addition, fructose dramatically slows fat burning and therefore causes weight gain. It elevates the presence of triglycerides along with LDL cholesterol. Research shows that it doesn't cause insulin production. As a result, after consumption, a person may not feel full, and so many people may eat more than they should. Chromium levels can be lowered by this sweetener, which then prompts sugar cravings. This can be a big contributing factor in type 2 diabetes. The tragedy is that because of its low glycemic index (GI), fructose was recommended for diabetics for many years, which made their health much worse.

Though fructose has a GI of 19, it does increase blood fructose, which is much worse. This can cause much more cell damage than glucose, because it binds to cellular proteins much more quickly than glucose does. This causes a release of large numbers of oxygen radicals like hydrogen peroxide, which kills everything in sight. One twenty-ounce soda produces a serum fructose concentration of six micromolars, enough to do major arterial and pancreatic damage. A micromolar is a measure of amount-of-substance concentration.[8] Dr. Lustig says, "Fructose's poisonous effects have nothing to do with glycaemic index; they are beyond glycaemic index."[9]

Avoid products that list on the label fructose, high-fructose corn syrup, honey (usually it's not pure honey and certainly not local and unprocessed), fruit juice concentrate, or corn syrup solids—all contain fructose. Watch out for bacon, hot dogs, sausages, and cold cuts, which typically contain variations of fructose, along with soups, sauces, gravies, snacks, commercial beverages, baby foods, ethnic foods, and fast food.

Maltodextrin

Maltodextrin is derived from plants, which is why it's often called "natural," but it's highly processed, making it anything but natural. Maltodextrin is most often made from GMO corn, rice, or potato starch, or it may come from wheat. The starch is then cooked and acids or enzymes are added to break it down, finally producing a white powder with a slightly sweet taste. Because it is cheap, malto-dextrin is often used as a thickener or a filler of manufactured foods. With a glycemic index of 100, you'll want to avoid it completely, so watch out for it on product labels, especially for the following foods:

- Canned fruits
- Desserts
- Instant puddings and gelatins
- Sauces
- Salad dressings
- Snacks
- Powdered drinks
- Packaged foods with sugar substitutes

Maltose

Maltose is also known as maltobiose, or malt sugar, and it is produced by the combination of two units of glucose, which results in starch. Maltose is used when fermenting barley, and it can also be used in beer brewing. When a third unit of glucose is added, maltotriose is formed, and adding even more glucose units produces maltodextrin. These various steps create concentrations of a sweetener that is often used in a number of different food products, including molasses and beer. Incidentally, maltose is also formed in the first step of the digestion of starchy foods; it's then broken down into glucose. Though about half as sweet as table sugar, it has a glycemic index of 105. Completely avoid it.

Trehalose

Trehalose is a compound composed of two sugars—both are glucose. It is stable both in high temperatures and under acidic conditions, but it also can act as an antioxidant. It's only about half as sweet as glucose, but in the body, enzymes break it down to glucose. Trehalose protects commercial food products that contain it from extreme temperatures or from drying out. Trehalose also preserves the texture and structure of frozen fruits and vegetables, and it is used to thicken purees and fillings and to enhance dried fruit flavors. It should be avoided.

Golden syrup

Golden syrup, or light treacle, is a thick, amber-colored form of inverted sugar syrup made by refining sugarcane or sugar beet juice into sugar or by treating a sugar solution with acid.

Modified sugar

Over half of the sugar in the United States is produced from sugar beets—and about half of those beets come from genetically modified (GM) plants. Unfortunately, modified sugar can be found in many of our premade foods, even savory and seemingly "healthy" products like soup and bread. With no requirements in our country that genetically modified foods be labeled at this time, you may be consuming a great deal more modified sugar than you think you are. I'd say to avoid it like a root canal, but without labeling, how will you know it's there?

Inverted sugar

Inverted sugar syrup combines glucose and fructose by splitting sucrose. The result, inverted sugar, is sweeter than sucrose. Those products that contain it retain moisture much better, and they are less prone to crystallization, which makes inverted sugar a product that is coveted by bakers. It is similar to high-fructose corn syrup.

Agave syrup

Traditional agave is made from boiled sap of the blue agave plant. Modern agave syrup is typically found in health food store products. Agave contains more fructose than glucose, which allows it to have a low glycemic index score. It is made up of 90 percent fructose; therefore it is not a good choice—for all the reasons that we have already discussed earlier regarding fructose, including scarring of the liver.

Fructose occurs naturally in fruits and some vegetables, but it is present there in small amounts. In each fruit or vegetable, it is also part of a complex of fiber, fatty acids, vitamins, and minerals. Natural fructose in whole foods is usually digested and absorbed slowly, but in its concentrated form, like agave, it is quickly digested and immediately absorbed into the bloodstream. From there it goes straight to the liver, and therefore has been linked to liver problems. According to Dr. Sarah Cimperman, "A 2008 study found that people who consume it regularly have a two- to three-fold higher risk of developing non-alcoholic fatty liver disease (NAFLD) compared to adults of similar age, gender and body mass index."[10]

Dr. Cimperman continues, "A 2010 study from Duke University Medical Center found that fructose consumption in people with NAFLD can cause hardening and scarring of the liver which may lead to cirrhosis, liver failure, liver cancer and the need for a liver transplant."[11] Completely avoid this "once darling" of the sweetener world.

Sorbitol

Sorbitol is a sugar alcohol that is produced from the corn sugar dextrose. It is used in chewing gum, "sugar-free candy," toothpaste, and shaving cream as a water-soluble bulking agent. I recommend that you avoid it because most of the corn is genetically modified.

Sweet Poison

Aspartame

This artificial sweetener is marketed under the names NutraSweet, Equal, NatraTaste, and Sugar Twin brands. It comes in the baby-blue packets and is found in diet or "sugar-free" foods and beverages. It's neither a diet sweetener nor a safe sugar-free option.

Research shows that artificial sweeteners such as aspartame lower appetite suppressant chemicals and encourage sugar cravings and sugar dependence, thereby raising the odds of weight gain. It has also been found to cause headaches, seizures, and heart palpitations. Brain tumors spiked when this sweetener entered the market. Top aspartame researchers also warn that aspartame consumption may be a contributing factor in skyrocketing autism rates, by way of methanol toxicity.[12]

Listen up! Research shows that aspartame worsens insulin sensitivity even more than refined sugar. This artificial sweetener promotes weight gain by tricking the body into thinking it will receive calories from sugar. When the calories don't arrive, carb cravings result and we want to eat more carbs; then we gain weight. It also disrupts our intestinal microflora, thereby raising our risk of both obesity and diabetes.[13]

ONE WOMAN'S ASPARTAME STORY

In October of 2001, my sister started getting very sick. She had stomach spasms, and she was having a hard time getting around. Walking was a major chore. It took everything she had just to get out of bed; she was in so much pain. By March 2002 she had undergone several tissue and muscle biopsies and was on twenty-four various prescription medications. The doctors could not determine what was wrong with her. She was in so much pain, and so sick. She just knew she was dying. She put her house, bank accounts, life insurance, etc., in her oldest daughter's name, and made sure that her younger children would be taken care of. She also wanted a last "hoorah," so she planned a trip to Florida (basically in a wheelchair) for March 22. On March 19 I called her to ask how her most recent tests went, and she said they didn't find anything on the test, but they believed she had MS. I recalled an article a friend of mine e-mailed to me, and I asked my sister if she drank diet soda. She told me that she did. As a matter of fact, she was getting ready to crack one open that moment. I told her not to open it, and to stop drinking the diet soda! I e-mailed her the article my friend, a lawyer, had sent.

My sister called me within thirty-two hours of our phone conversation and told me she had stopped drinking the diet soda *and* she could walk! The muscle spasms went away. She said she didn't feel 100 percent, but she sure felt a lot better. She told me she was going to her doctor with this article and would call me when she got home. Well, she called me, and said her doctor was amazed! He is going to call all of his MS patients to find out if they consumed artificial sweeteners of any kind.

In a nutshell, she was being poisoned by the aspartame in the diet soda and was literally dying a slow and miserable death. When she got to Florida on March 22, all she had to take was one pill, and that was a pill for the aspartame poisoning! She is well on her way to a complete recovery, and she is walking—no wheelchair. (An article about aspartame dangers) saved her life. If it says "sugar free" on the label, DO NOT EVEN THINK ABOUT IT![14]

Sucralose

Ah, those little yellow packets. Splenda! It's the trade name for sucralose—the no-calorie sugar substitute that took the world by storm a few years back. Here is its chemical composition: 1,6-Dichloro-1,6-dideoxy-β-D-fructofuranosyl-4-chloro-4-deoxy-α-D-galactopyranoside. How about those chemicals? Is that something you want to load your body up with? Splenda can be found in a wide variety of commercial foods and beverages. It has been advertised as a healthier choice than NutraSweet, and experts thought it was safe—for a while, that is. But new, scary findings say otherwise.

According to a research review published in the *Journal of Toxicology and Environmental Health*, Splenda can cause harmful effects in your body.[15] When you bake with it, potential toxic compounds called chloroproanols are released.[16] "Sucralose can alter insulin responses and blood sugar levels, has been associated with inflammatory bowel disease, and may even alter genes, the researchers note."[17] It's associated with many of the same adverse effects as aspartame, including headaches, seizures, heart palpitations, and weight gain.[18] Splenda also reduces beneficial gut bacteria by 50 percent.[19] Disrupting your intestinal microflora is one of the many mechanisms by which artificial sweeteners, including saccharin and aspartame, cause obesity and diabetes.[20] It's a poisonous substitute for sugar. You're better off with sugar if you had only two choices. But thankfully you have many healthier choices.

Saccharin

Then there are the pretty pink packets. Popular brand names of saccharin include Sweet'N Low, Sweet Twin, and Necta Sweet. It is two hundred to seven hundred times sweeter than table sugar. A few studies with rats showed that they suffered from bladder cancer after consuming saccharin. Although this has not appeared in human studies, the concern is still there. If something causes cancer in rats, long-term effects on humans are of concern. Saccharin is part of the group of sulfonamides, which can cause allergic reactions in some individuals. Commonly reported reactions to saccharin use in some individuals include headaches, diarrhea, skin issues, and headaches.

Sweeteners to Limit

These are not "bad boy" sweeteners, but they should be used in small amounts. They are still sugar.

Erythritol and Mannitol

Although these sugar alcohols may not produce blood sugar spikes and they may have half the calories of sugar (including sucrose, glucose, and fructose), erythritol and mannitol are still sweeteners to limit. Erythritol is frequently produced from plant sugars, then mixed with water, and fermented with a natural culture. After it is filtered and crystallized, it is then dried. The final product comes in the form of white granules, or powder, and it looks and tastes just like sugar. You can replace 1 cup white sugar with 1 1/4 cup erythritol in your recipes. In reasonable amounts, erythritol doesn't cause diarrhea and digestive upset the way other sugar alcohols, like sorbitol and xylitol, have been known to cause.

In contrast, mannitol is usually produced from seaweed, using ethanol, water, and methanol to steam and hydrolyze this crude material. Mannitol is then recrystallized from the extracted product that resulted from this process. This sugar alcohol is often used in both food and pharmaceutical products. It is about 50 percent as sweet as sucrose and it has a desirable cooling effect. It may be used to mask bitter tastes of medications or foods. Mannitol does not promote tooth decay and has a low caloric content.

Xylitol

Xylitol is produced from either birch tree bark or waste products from the pulp industry. I only recommend xylitol that is made from birch bark; avoid the rest. Xylitol may be used in equal amounts as a substitute for sugar. Because it is slightly sweeter than sugar, you can get by with a little less xylitol. Replace 1 cup white sugar with 3/4 cup and 1 tablespoon xylitol. This sweetener has a very low glycemic index and 40 percent fewer calories than sugar. It has been recommended by dentists for use in toothpaste because it also has antibacterial properties.

Molasses

As many people know, molasses is a thick, dark syrup, and today it is primarily a by-product of sugar production from sugarcane or sugar beets. Beet molasses can be very bitter and is frequently used in animal feed. Sucrose is predominant in sugarcane molasses, along with small amounts of glucose and fructose. Molasses is not quite as sweet as table sugar; it can be purchased in three grades:

sulfured, unsulfured, and blackstrap. Molasses is actually made with sulfur to process unripe green sugarcane. This chemical is not good for humans to ingest. Unsulfured molasses is unripened sugarcane processed without sulfur, making this grade a better choice for our diets. The third grade is made by boiling in order to extract table sugar from sugarcane, which produces a thick, dark syrup known as blackstrap molasses. This type is the richest in nutrients—especially calcium, magnesium, potassium, and iron, along with small amounts of copper and selenium. When molasses is processed from cane juice without high heat, it may contain trace active enzymes. Blackstrap molasses is not as sweet as sugar, and it has a glycemic index of 55.

Sorghum

In some regions of the United States, sweet sorghum syrup is sometimes called molasses, or sorghum molasses. Often confused with true molasses, sorghum is actually made from the sorghum plant, a cereal grass that is more golden in color. Sweet sorghum is a thick syrup with a GI of 50, which resembles molasses in appearance and texture. African slaves originally introduced sorghum to the United States, and even today it is a common ingredient in many soul-food recipes. Unsulfured blackstrap molasses is a good substitute for sorghum.

Date Sugar

Date sugar is usually considered a natural sweetener because it is not processed. It is made by powdering or grinding up chopped, dried dates. Date sugar is light brown in color and is comprised of 40 percent sucrose, 30 percent glucose, and 30 percent fructose. It has a very sweet taste but a grainy texture. It can be used for baking if melting the sugar is not required. One cup of refined sugar can be replaced by about two-thirds cup of date sugar. Date sugar appears as tiny brown specks in many baked goods. It contains calcium, iron, magnesium, phosphorus, zinc, copper, manganese, and selenium. However, it may cause a sudden spike in blood sugar, so people with sugar metabolism challenges should avoid it.

Honey

Bees produce honey from the nectar of flowers. True raw honey that is not heated to more than 118 degrees is loaded with active enzymes, vitamins, phytonutrients, and many minerals. Raw honey is often used as a remedy for sore throats because it does have some antibacterial and disinfectant properties. However, true raw honey is not so easy to find; you'll have the best chance of finding it at local farmers markets, co-ops, directly from local beekeepers, or off the Internet. Most of what you find in stores, even health stores, has been pasteurized. The more processed the honey, the fewer nutrients it has. Also, be aware that not all bees are raised the same. Many beekeepers feed their bees antibiotic-laced sugar and sugar syrups. This is very destructive to the health of the bees and the honey they produce.

Even worse, however, *Food Safety News* has reported that "honey banned as unsafe in dozens of countries [is] being imported and sold here in record quantities." Their investigation found that about one-third or more of all honey comes from China. The practice is known as honey laundering. This honey can be tainted with illegal antibiotics, including chloramphenicol, along with heavy metals like lead.[21]

Be aware that there is also "fake honey." According to *Food*

Safety News: "[A] favorite con among Chinese brokers was to mix sugar water, malt sweeteners, corn or rice syrup, jaggery [traditional non-centrifugal cane sugar], barley malt sweetener or other additives with a bit of actual honey. In recent years, many shippers have eliminated the honey completely and just use thickened, colored, natural or chemical sweeteners labeled as honey."[22]

Buy only raw organic honey from local growers. Besides more nutrients and less contamination, raw honey produced in your local area is believed to help improve the body's immune response to local allergens.

Honey consists of the same simple sugars as table sugar—half fructose and half glucose. It is more than twice as sweet as refined sugar, with more calories. Replace 2 cups sugar with 3/4 cup honey, and reduce liquids by 2 to 4 tablespoons. Because honey is more acidic than sugar, you may want to add a pinch of baking soda to neutralize it. You will also need to reduce the cooking temperature by 25 degrees.

With a higher glycemic index than table sugar, honey is not a good choice for people with sugar metabolism challenges.

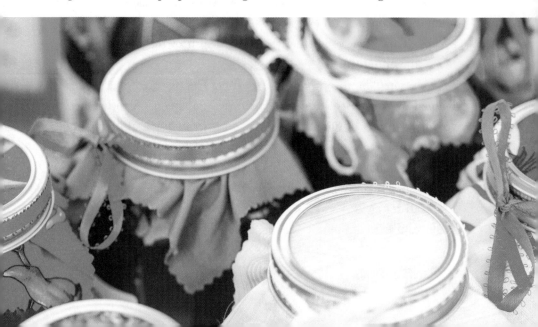

WHAT IS KILLING THE HONEYBEES?

According to an article in *E/The Environmental Magazine*, the increased use of pesticides and herbicides, often ingested by honeybees during the pollination process, may be primarily responsible for the collapse of many bee colonies. The article states, "Commercial beehives are also subjected to direct chemical fumigation at regular intervals to ward off destructive mites."[23] Genetically modified crops (GMOs) that are generating pollen with compromised nutritional values are also suspect.[24] It is possible that a buildup of both adverse chemicals and genetically modified crop pollen has brought about the "tipping point" for bees, stressing their populations to the point of collapse.[25] "The 98 pesticides and metabolites detected in mixtures up to 214 ppm (parts per million) in bee pollen alone represents a remarkably high level for toxicants in the brood and adult food of this primary pollinator," said researcher Christopher Mullin and his colleagues in the journal Public Library of Science-One.[26]

According to the Organic Consumers Association, "organic bee colonies, where chemicals and genetically modified crops are avoided, are not experiencing the same kind of catastrophic collapses."[27] The article in *E* continues, "Bee populations may also be vulnerable to other factors, such as the recent increase in atmospheric electromagnetic radiation as a result of growing numbers of cell phones and wireless communication towers." Unfortunately, this may interfere with the bees' ability to navigate.[28] According to *E*, "A small study at Germany's Landau University found that bees would not return to their hives when mobile phones were placed nearby. Further research is currently underway in the US to determine the extent of such radiation-related phenomena on bees and other insect populations."[29] In addition, bees are being bred and

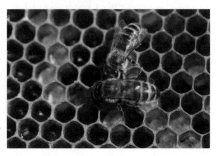

raised to survive a shorter off-season, in order for them to be ready to pollinate as soon as the almond tree bloom begins in February. This practice, while perhaps beneficial to human honey producers, could unfortunately be lowering the bees' immunity to viruses.

As the bees have begun to die off at an alarmingly rapid rate, scientists are beginning to worry about what we will do to pollinate our crops should they become extinct. The sober truth is that without bees to pollinate our world, we will not have food. A 2007 *New York Times* article states, "A Cornell University study has estimated that honeybees annually pollinate more than $14 billion worth of seeds and crops in the United States, mostly fruits, vegetables and nuts. 'Every third bite we consume in our diet is dependent on a honeybee to pollinate that food,' said Zac Browning, vice president of the American Beekeeping Federation."[30]

For example, beekeepers in many Southern states will truck their bees north in the spring to assist blueberry or cranberry growers. Almonds, apples, soybeans, and strawberries—as well as meat from animals that feed on pollinated crops—will likely become much more expensive if there is a shortage of bees to pollinate the trees and vines. Even worse, honeybees are an indicator species, like the canary in the coal mine, so what does this indicate for the rest of us who share the planet?[31]

Pure Maple Syrup

Maple syrup is obtained by tapping sap from sugar maple trees. It is then concentrated by boiling until most of the water has evaporated. The boiling process denatures enzymes. It comes in two grades: grade A (often used as pancake syrup) and grade B (usually used for baking). Maple syrup is about twice as sweet as sugar, so you need less: replace 1 cup sugar with 1/2 to 2/3 cup maple syrup. Though maple syrup provides many nutrients, it has a similar glycemic index to table sugar, and therefore should be used in moderation.

Not all maple syrup labeled "pure" is truly pure or sustainable. Only organically certified indicates that no chemicals were used to manage the forest, and that no formaldehyde was used in tapping the trees. Formaldehyde slows the natural closing of the tap holes.

Brown Rice Syrup

Brown rice syrup is made by adding enzymes to cooked rice to break down the starches into smaller sugars. Next, impurities are filtered out and excess water is evaporated to thicken it into a syrup. It's made up of three sugars: maltotriose (52 percent), maltose (45 percent), and glucose (3 percent), with maltose consisting of two glucose molecules, and maltotriose consisting of three glucose molecules. Brown rice syrup has a glycemic index of 98 and raises blood sugar levels. It can be found in a number of health food store products such as dairy-free ice creams, but it is not a great choice. Use this sweetener very sparingly.

Coconut Palm Sugar and Syrup

Coconut palm sugar is made from the nectar of the coconut tree (not the palm tree). Once collected, it is boiled and processed into granules. Coconut palm sugar is low on the glycemic index, which has benefits when it comes to glucose and lipid levels in people with diabetes. The major component of coconut sugar is sucrose (70 to 79 percent) followed by glucose and fructose (3 to 9 percent) each. Coconut palm sugar has a higher nutritional content than most other sweeteners. It is especially rich in potassium, magnesium, zinc, and iron. It has a low glycemic index of 35 and has been shown to cause fewer blood sugar spikes. You can substitute it for sugar in equal parts.

Be aware that some coconut palm sugar is mixed with cane sugar and other malt-based ingredients such as maltodextrin. Look for pure coconut palm sugar or coconut nectar with nothing added.

Best Sweetener Choices

Stevia

Stevia is a zero-calorie sweetener made from a substance called stevioside that is found in the leaves of the stevia plant. Unlike artificial sweeteners, stevia is actually a healthy no-calorie choice! It is very low on the glycemic index scale, and it may improve insulin sensitivity. This makes it a great choice for diabetics and for people who are insulin-resistant. Stevia can be found in green packets in some establishments and is available in a variety of forms:

- Powdered dried herb (green color)
- Liquid extract
- Refined crystals (white)
- Refined crystals mixed with inulin or other fiber as a bulking agent

The powdered dried herb contains beneficial nutrients, but it can have a slightly undesirable aftertaste. However, the liquid extract is delicious, especially in recipes calling for brown sugar, molasses, or honey. I like the vanilla crème–flavored one.

Stevia is very sweet (two hundred to three hundred times sweeter than cane sugar). When converting a recipe from sugar to stevia, use about ½ teaspoon stevia extract for each cup of sugar.

Barley Malt Syrup

Barley malt syrup is a natural sweetener produced from sprouted barley. The process involves sprouting, and then the sprouted barley is dried quickly. It's cooked slowly until a sweet, dark syrup forms, which is half as sweet as white sugar and looks very similar to molasses. Then it is filtered to remove impurities and bottled or dried and made into powder. Barley malt syrup consists of 65 percent maltose, 30 percent complex carbohydrates, and 3 percent protein. Because it doesn't contain fructose, it is considered less detrimental to the body and does not cause blood sugar spikes.

Luo Han Guo

In many Western countries, Luo Han Guo is known as "monk fruit." It is a natural zero-calorie sweetener that has been used in China and the East for over eight hundred years. It contains many antioxidants and has often been used for medicinal purposes. Its sweetness comes from mogrosides, which make up about 1 percent of this fruit by weight. But it is about three hundred times as sweet as sugar with a zero glycemic index, making it suitable for diabetics.

Chapter 9

THE TEN-STEP SUGAR DETOX PLAN: HOW TO FORCE SUGAR TO THROW IN THE TOWEL

I**T'S TIME TO** get rid of your sweet tooth *now*! You could be just a few days away from a healthier, happier you. You'll enjoy your journey much more without sugar. Trust me. I know. Having gone from sick all the time to feeling fantastic most days of my life, with energy and a "no fog" brain, I want everyone to share this wonderful experience of true health and well-being. You truly can get rid of bloating, gas, reflux, irritable bowel, joint or muscle pain, brain fog, memory or mood problems, sinus problems, and allergy symptoms. And you can lose weight easily when you ditch the sugar and refined carbs. It's all one detox plan away.

By now you know from all the research presented in preceding chapters how detrimental sugar is for your body. So here you are now at the chapter where you actually get to give the stuff up. How do you feel about that? Are you excited? Scared? Wondering what you'll do when you're tempted? I've been there through it all and survived—actually thrived. I know you can too. I'm going to help you reach your goals and give sugar the knockout punch. It's time for you to be sugar free, healthy, and whole.

Basic Steps to Get Started

- **Make a decision and commitment to detox from sugar.** You must be committed to this program 100 percent or you'll cheat and eventually throw in the towel. You must want to be sugar free more than you want the momentary little sweet pleasure or "high."

- **Pick the right day to start.** Choose a day to begin when you don't have someone's birthday party to attend or a celebration dinner. You'll eventually develop the willpower to navigate through special events, but it's not a good idea to start on a day with one planned.

- **Go cold turkey.** The only way to stop something like sugar is to stop it completely. Easing in doesn't work with something as addictive as cocaine and heroin. If you eat a little bit less to ease into it, you'll keep getting triggered to want more sweets. You've got to stop it all and not look back. This is the way to handle a sugar habit; completely let it go. Get online and download the song "Let It Go" from the movie *Frozen*. Sing along at the top of your lungs. Now is the time to reset your body's neurotransmitters and hormones. You can quit all forms of sugar, flour products, and all artificial sweeteners, all of which cause increased sugar and carb cravings, slow down your metabolism, and lead to fat storage. Avoid as much as possible foods that come in boxes, packages, or cans so you can avoid all the hidden sugars. Also, give up grains and white potatoes for thirty days as well. They turn to sugar more readily than other foods. Eat real, whole, fresh food.

- **Scrutinize every label.** It's time to root out sugar in all its forms. Remember manufacturers want to sneak it past your watchful eyes. Well, no more. Having read chapter 8, "The Sugar Shopping Guide," you are now an informed shopper. And when you're just not sure whether something is sugar or not, flip through your "Sugar Shopping Guide" to help identify those sneaky additions. If you can't find the name, don't buy the product. Remember manufacturers keep coming up with new disguises.

- **Make emergency snack packs.** Don't get caught without good food. Whether you're traveling, shopping, or at work, it's not wise to get stuck with only fast food or vending machine choices. Make up emergency snack packs to take with you. They could contain things like nuts and seeds, unsweetened coconut flakes, nut butter and veggie sticks, turkey jerky, or an apple with a seed butter.

- **Get inflammation under control.** My recent book *The Juice Lady's Anti-Inflammation Diet* is all about getting inflammation under control. Studies have shown that inflammation can trigger blood sugar imbalances, insulin resistance, prediabetes, and even type 2 diabetes.[1] The most common foods that cause inflammation include sugar, artificial sweeteners, junk food, refined flour, soda, coffee, black tea, alcohol, unhealthy oils, and trans fats. Food sensitivities to gluten and dairy bring about inflammation if these foods are consumed, but we often crave the very foods we're allergic to. Without them, we feel crummy and we crave even more of them to stop the symptoms. You should quit gluten, sugar, and dairy for ten days and see if you feel better. Get the inflammatory foods out of your diet, and you'll immediately experience renewed energy, relief from cravings, and freedom from many negative symptoms and the healing of illness.

- **Exercise.** Working out helps you improve insulin resistance. Work out with weights for at least part of your routine and you'll build more muscle. This will help you burn more calories even at a resting heart rate and help in maintaining balanced blood sugar. Morning is the best time to get moving. It's a great head start on your day.

- **Get some sun.** Sun exposure helps balance insulin and blood glucose levels. It also helps your serotonin level; hence you have a better mood. Hopefully then you won't go running for sweets to prop up your flagging emotions.

- **Scare yourself into going sugar free.** Take a look at the story aired by *60 Minutes* entitled "Is Sugar Toxic?" This is a life-changing report for anyone who needs a nudge to kick the sugar habit. Then do what I do. Look at sugar like you look at poison. Rat poison is sweet; in fact, it tastes so good that ten thousand toddlers are endangered each year from ingesting it. I look at everything with sugar like it was rat poison. It is poison. If you see it as that, no matter how pretty it is dressed up in a dessert, you won't be tempted in the slightest. I look at desserts now, and they look disgusting. I hope you can get there too.

- **De-stress; learn to live from a happy heart.** When you are stressed out, your hormones get out of whack. Cortisol shoots up, and you get hungry, but you rarely crave salmon and veggies at such a time. Cortisol causes belly fat storage and leads to type 2 diabetes. My husband teaches this class at our retreats and uses biofeedback and uses the emWave to help people measure their stress. It involves deep breathing. Taking deep breaths is said to activate your vagus nerve, which can shift your metabolism from fat storage to fat burning. It can quickly move you out of a stressful state to a state of coherence. Take a long, deep breath in to the count of five, hold, and then let it out to a count of five. Do this five times whenever you feel stress coming on or when it is full-blown. You can also try it before a meal.

- **Let go of hurts, grudges, and negative emotions.** Such emotions and thoughts can keep us hostage to unpleasant memories. We can get trapped in the cogs of such wheels and keep turning to sweets for solace. It's time to let it all go. Let it go!" You'll know when you do. You'll feel a shift in your soul.

- **When you stumble, get back in the race.** We all have times when we eat things we know we shouldn't. Sugar seems to have the biggest lure for many of us. The important thing to remember is when you fall in the "sugar ditch" that you get right back out. Don't say you've blown it so you may as well just go for the gusto and enjoy your sweets. Rather, get right back on track.

JUDY'S GETTING BACK ON TRACK

I had a harder time this go-round. I went back to some of my old ways and had a fling with sugar. It's pleasurable for the moment, but when the effects wore off, I found myself in that same old pit. Since beginning your program (Jumpstart Health & Fitness) in June 2014, I had been lifted from that pit and had forgotten what it was like to live chained to sugar. Juicing and cooking from scratch has been a big effort for me, but after crawling after the sugar bowl, I think I'd rather push the restart button, get back in the race, and run for the prize.

Being off the sugar habit (not 100 percent sugar-free yet, there are occasional times when I eat sugar, but not often or habitually), the main thing I've noticed has been in my thinking. Brooding and obsessively replaying unpleasant things in my mind has stopped. My diet had been heavy in sugar/fat/flour combinations (cookies, doughnuts, pastries, etc.). Hurts turned to long-term grudges, with my mind being on a hamster wheel over things. I would forgive over and over and over, really confused as to why I wasn't getting over things. When I swapped out the sugar for juicing, the obsessing stopped. When I was a child, I didn't have a diet heavy in sugar. I wasn't easily offended, was able to look into situations with understanding, and not take things personally. Now that I've eliminated sugar as much as possible, I more easily take things in stride. When something happens, my mind doesn't latch on to it as it had before. Now, when I do find myself camped out over something, I know I have to do my part to make things right. It's more problem-solving, rather than trying to untangle a snarly, emotional mess.

Here's another unexpected benefit. I've been off sugar about six months. I recently noticed I'm losing the high I would get when out shopping. I'm not stirred up inside by the rising/falling blood sugar levels. I'm not as impulsive as I used to be. I'm better at waiting or not getting (something) at all. I always stayed within my budget, but it's nice not to have that ruling over me the way it did. When the weather warms up, I believe I'll be looking for new and different things to do. I'm excited for spring in a way I've not known before.

—Judy

Giving Up Sugar—What to Expect

We all know something about comfort-food eating and carbohydrates. The brain gets addicted to sweet comfort. When you run on higher blood sugar levels, the body gets used to its stimulating release of happy mood neurotransmitters such as gamma-aminobutyric acid (GABA), dopamine, and serotonin. These neurotransmitters for the most part have a calming effect, although serotonin and dopamine can be stimulating at times. The second challenge is our set point for blood sugar (a measure against which blood sugar levels are compared and controlled). It is speculated that with long-term consumption of sweets, this is set higher, if blood sugar runs consistently high. For example, there are people with diabetes who run consistently high blood sugar levels but feel hypoglycemic if their blood sugars drop to what would be considered normal blood sugar levels. If this is you, be aware of your set point issues and how to deal with hypoglycemia symptoms. Protein is key here.

TARGET BLOODSUGAR LEVELS

- On waking up (before breakfast): 80 to 120 mg/dL (80–90 is ideal)
- Before meals: 80 to 120 mg/dL (80–90 is ideal)
- 2 hours after meals: 160 or less mg/dL
- At bedtime: 100 to 140 mg/dL

I've worked with people who say it's too hard to give up sweets because there is an unpleasant period of transition time. First of all, take it from one who knows, *it's worth it all*. I want to give you some idea of what kinds of symptoms you might experience. I also want to let you know how to minimize symptoms and move through the transition period with greater ease.

Impulse Control Challenges

Depending on how long you've been eating sweets, breaking this habit may come with some challenges. It's one of the reasons people struggle to change their relationship with sugar. There is the desire and longing to change, but the day-to-day practice can feel like it's beyond reach. What about you? When you're hungry, do you feel overwhelmed? Are you unable to overcome triggers and impulses like the urge to eat cookies, doughnuts, or ice cream? Do you feel lost without your old friend sugar or bread? You have an inner wisdom about what to eat, but it is often lost or overwhelmed with the addiction to sweets and/or refined carbs. Now is the time to honestly face your challenges with impulse control. It's time to ask for help if you need it. You can determine you'll make the changes necessary to overcome your impulse control challenges.

Symptoms That May Manifest When You Quit Sugar

Please don't get scared if you get a few symptoms. You are just detoxing from an addictive substance. You may get some of these symptoms. I've never met anyone who had them all. You may get none of them. If you do experience some symptoms, press on. You may feel sick for a few days, but don't give up. It's worth the journey. Here's what you might experience:

- Continually feeling hungry
- Headaches
- Dizziness
- Flu-like symptoms
- Crankiness or irritability
- Sleep disturbances
- Shakiness
- Weight loss (you're probably excited about that one!)
- Low energy, fatigue
- Mood swings
- Muscle aches and pains
- Nausea, vomiting, stomach cramps, diarrhea
- Faster heartbeat; higher or lower blood pressure
- Chills or sweating
- Cravings for sweets

How Long Will Detox Symptoms Last?

We are all different. Sugar withdrawal symptoms may be short-lived, almost nonexistent, or drag on a bit. The duration you experience will largely depend on you—your body chemistry, your level of detox, and how you detox. Some people can quickly adjust to functioning without sugar, while others may struggle to resist sugar cravings and the comfort or reward that they get when they have something sweet. It's unusual to experience nothing. Most people notice some sort of a withdrawal period after they ditch sugar, but the length of this withdrawal period varies. Some people report feeling considerably better right away. That's a great reward. By the fourth or fifth day of your sugar detox, your brain fog may begin to lift. After a week, your desire for sugar should be going away, and you should feel more in control. It may take a few weeks for your strong cravings to subside. Don't worry though; you'll get there. Some people are virtually withdrawal-symptom free within a few days, while it can take others close to a month to feel completely normal and completely detoxed from sugar.

You may have sugar-detox symptoms for a variety of reasons. If you have an overgrowth of yeast known as *Candida albicans*, you'll get some die-off when you stop eating sweets, flour products, and starchy foods. That can cause symptoms and cravings. Products like caffeine, alcohol, and sugar cause dopamine deficiency in the brain, and low dopamine can contribute to detox symptoms. If your favorite form of sugar is a soda, flavored sweet coffee, or chocolate, you may actually get caffeine withdrawal symptoms too. And some people are just more sensitive and reactive than others.

If you've eaten sweets on a regular basis, the first forty-eight hours will usually be the toughest. You may be irritable, grouchy, or hungry for something you can't quite identify. But when you get the right amount of protein, fat, vegetables, and low-sugar fruit along with green smoothies and/or juices, you'll be fine. Actually you should gain energy, feel happier and empowered, and have a better sense of well-being. It's like the ultimate palate cleanse. You'll come to appreciate the taste of whole foods, like the subtle salty taste of celery, the gentle sweetness of blueberries, or the zing of a spice like ginger. Cutting out sweets can help crush sugar cravings and reboot your brain. You really can enjoy foods that are not sweet. You'll find you don't have to have something sweet after dinner. By the third day, your taste buds should be happy campers with a crisp apple.

Detoxing from sugar should help with fatigue. If your body is going to produce the energy that it needs, then your cells must be able to eliminate substances like lactic acid, which is a by-product of sugar metabolism. When you feel tired after a vigorous session of exercise, it is largely due to your body's inability to eliminate lactic acid and other metabolic waste fast enough after your workout. Your blood and lymph circulation can become sluggish, or your cell membranes can have such a poor electrical charge that you cannot properly eliminate the waste your body has produced. This causes people to feel fatigued and crave a "sugar fix" or a caffeine pickup to help with energy.

Helpful Hints for Withdrawal Symptoms

1. Drink plenty of water; it helps flush out metabolic waste and toxins.

2. Make sure you don't get constipated to prevent headaches and other withdrawal symptoms.

3. Make more time for sleep; your body is changing and detoxing. You may need more rest.

4. Exercise daily to spark up energy.

5. When you're hungry or craving sweets, eat some protein, such as cooked beans or a slice of organic turkey, along with a healthy source of fat, such as almonds, pecans, walnuts, or pumpkin seeds.

6. Take a combination of calcium citrate (500 mg) and magnesium citrate (250 mg) before bed, especially whenever you're irritable, restless, or have trouble sleeping.

7. Drink ginger or peppermint tea or make a vegetable juice with ginger for an upset stomach.

Sugar Detox Ten-Step Plan

Modify this program to make it work for you and your family's lifestyle. If you mess up, forgive yourself and jump right back in the race. But whatever you do, don't go back to your old diet and start eating sugar. My hope is that now that you are more educated, selective, and empowered, you'll stay the course and ditch the sugar for good.

Step 1: Avoid all sugar

For the first thirty days, avoid *all* forms of added sugar—both real and artificial, even healthy sweeteners. It takes about thirty days to create a new habit. It can take about this amount of time to reset your appetite, retrain your taste buds, and kiss your sugar cravings good-bye.

Avoid all artificial sweeteners. Even though sweeteners such as

Splenda, Equal, Sweet'N Low, and other zero-calorie sugar substitutes don't add any calories, they *do* overwhelm your taste buds with
"sweet," and then you want more and more. Your 10-step sugar detox
will be the ultimate reality check. It's a learning experience to open
your eyes to just how sugar has slipped into your daily life.

Get rid of all sweeteners in your house, car, and office. Clean
out your pantry. This step is very important. If you have sweet stuff
in your house, car, or office, you *will* get tempted. It's time to haul
out the trash (it literally is trash for the body). Clean out the freezer
and the fridge too. Here's the tricky part, though. If you live with
people who don't want to quit sugar, and who are not underage, you
may have to strengthen your willpower. With children you can start
a fun new way of eating with fresh fruit, smoothies, juices, and fun
healthy desserts made with stevia. But you'll still need to strengthen
your willpower. For the first thirty days, you need the ultimate palate
cleanse—nothing sweet at all, not even sweet fruit (just low-sugar
fruit like berries).

To break the cycle that triggers the brain into a sugar binge
attack, you need to get all sweeteners out of sight. Remember, sight
triggers the brain to want what it sees. It's too tempting when sweets
are lurking in the pantry. If you can't bear to throw them away, send
them on a vacation to a friend's house or donate them. This means
sugar, honey, maple syrup, agave nectar, and artificial sweetener.
The first thirty days, eat nothing sweet except for fresh fruit.

Ditch the liquid calories. Liquid sweetener is worse than
solid food with sugar or flour. It's more like mainlining sugar directly
to your liver, your fat storage machine. Unlike food, there isn't fiber
or fat attached that causes slower absorption. It's so easy to down
large amounts of soda, fruit juice, sports drinks, sweetened tea,
and syrupy coffee. One 20-ounce soda has 16 teaspoons of sugar.

Gatorade contains 9 teaspoons of the sweet stuff in one 20-ounce bottle. Avoid the energy drinks as well. Almost all of them contain artificial sweeteners and lots of caffeine. They can be dangerous. This year my schnauzer's groomer's stepdaughter died at the age of thirty-eight while drinking an energy drink and taking diet pills.

Step 2: Cut your caffeine intake

Small, occasional cups of coffee, the size of an old-fashioned china teacup, are fine. For some people, there may be some benefits of occasional use. But that's only if it's fresh, high-quality, low-acid, and organic. Conventional coffee beans are among the most pesticide-sprayed crops in the world. According to *The Christian Science Monitor*, "conventional farms apply as much as 250 pounds of chemical fertilizers on every acre"[2] Dr. Mercola states, "Pesticides contribute to a wide range of health problems, including prostate and other types of cancers, Parkinson's disease, and miscarriages in pregnant women."[3] Most people have far more than a small or occasional cup of high-quality coffee. We're into great big mugs of the stuff and Grande, Venti, or Trenta "Big Gulp" cups of coffee. We go for instant coffee because it's faster; even worse, we go for that murky brown stuff out of an office coffee machine or vending machine. This is anything but organic, good-quality, and small portioned. Commercially made coffee is rarely organic.

There are several other good reasons to ditch coffee. First off, coffee stimulates the production of hydrochloric acid (HCl). HCl should only be produced to digest meals, and if your body is making HCl too often in response to coffee, it may then not have the ability to produce enough HCl when it comes time to deal with a big meal. Protein digestion particularly is affected by an HCl deficiency in the stomach. If you have drunk too much coffee and thus cannot digest protein properly, this can contribute to acid reflux (GERD), often caused by low stomach acid. Unfortunately at that point many people take antacids, which are about the worst thing they could take if they have low stomach acid!

Coffee also causes further acid reflux and heartburn because it relaxes the lower esophageal sphincter. This small muscle is intended to remain tightly closed when you eat, to prevent the contents of your stomach from splashing back into the esophagus and burning its delicate lining. However, even drinking decaf coffee regularly causes heartburn problems for some people; this is likely due to the other compounds in coffee that contribute to acid reflux.

Finally, drinking coffee for energy can actually create a jittery tension in your body that will make it difficult to relax. Just one cup of coffee can also "turn on" your stress hormones, which can then interfere with the digestive process as well as put you in a "fight or flight" response. This can cause you to crave simple carbohydrates for fuel so you can fight or run from the enemy. But we don't usually run today because we don't actually have a tiger or a bear chasing us, so all those carbs don't get burned up—they just turn to fat.

3. Skip the foods that turn to sugar easily

The fast-burning foods like white flour products turn to sugar quickly. Avoid wheat and other grains, alcohol, and starchy foods like white potatoes. Not everyone is addicted to sweets. Some people crave bread, pasta, or mashed potatoes. Or maybe it's crackers, granola, or white rice for you. Be aware of sneaky sources of sugar like tomato-based sauces, salad dressings, and marinades. Minimize dairy due to lactose (milk sugar).

You want to eat mostly slow-burning foods—protein, fats, and complex carbohydrates such as vegetables. This is not to say that you can't have a scoop of mashed potatoes once in a while or some white rice. As was mentioned earlier, white rice and sugar are metabolized differently; therefore, the starches are not nearly as bad as the sugars. But make the majority of your food slow-burning foods that take a long time to digest. These foods curb the sugar cravings because they provide a steady release of calories into your bloodstream versus a flood all at once. Fast-burning carbs like white bread, sugar, fruit juice, and pasta spike up glucose in your bloodstream quickly. This causes an excessive spike in insulin, leading to wide swings in blood sugar and setting you up for fat storage and sugar cravings. Your body also can't burn a huge caloric load for energy, so it increases the fat storage hormones and voilà—you store more fat. These fast-burning foods also cause "toxic hunger"—symptoms triggered when your glucose is at its lowest, which will send you scavenging for more sweets soon after you've finished eating those fast-burners.

4. Include plenty of fresh vegetable juice and/or green smoothies

These super foods offer your body superior nutrition. Have at least one fresh vegetable juice or green smoothie each day. If you can find wheatgrass juice, it will help you immensely. Wheatgrass is the queen of alkalizing drinks. Alkalizing is so important. Sugar is highly acidic. It's time to flush out acids with alkalizing food. According to the Mayo Clinic, "Wheatgrass provides a concentrated amount of nutrients, including iron; calcium; magnesium; amino acids; chlorophyll; and vitamins A, C and E."[4] When your body is well fed, you have fewer cravings. This makes it much easier to give up sugar. If you can't find or make fresh wheatgrass juice, I have found a wheatgrass juice powder that is the next best thing. Check it out in the resource guide (see Appendix).

WHEATGRASS JUICE (OR DEHYDRATED WHEATGRASS JUICE CAPSULES)

I just wanted to thank you for recommending that your readers add Wheatgrass/Sweet Wheat to their diet. I'm forty years old and was worried that I was going to be in a brain fog for the rest of my life. Well, thankfully after starting my Sweet Wheat regimen, I have been able to focus at work and have lost my appetite for sweets. Thank you again for providing us with such excellent and unbiased information.

—E

5. Power up with protein

Protein is a key to balancing blood sugar and insulin and cutting cravings. Start your day with cage-free, organic farm eggs or a protein shake. Use nuts, seeds, eggs, fish, chicken, or grass-fed meat during the day. One serving size of animal protein should be 4 to 6 ounces, which is about the size of your palm. Choose only clean sources of protein—free-range organic poultry and eggs, and grass-fed meat—to avoid the antibiotics and hormones given to factory farm animals.

6. Eat your veggies

That's the non-starchy ones in particular, which include greens, the cruciferous family (cauliflower, broccoli, brussels sprouts, kale, and collards), asparagus, green beans, mushrooms, onions, zucchini, tomatoes, fennel, eggplant, artichokes, and peppers. These are the complex carbs. Organic is always best, but if you can't afford all organic, at least avoid the ones on the Dirty Dozen list. You can always view the list of the Dirty Dozen and the Clean Fifteen at www.ewg.org. For the first thirty days, avoid white potatoes as much as possible.

7. Drink eight glasses of water a day

Consuming eight 8-ounce glasses of pure water daily is important for this process because it will keep your body well hydrated, can reduce headaches and constipation, and will flush toxins out of your system. This also helps get rid of metabolic waste and flushes the liver.

8. Supplement your diet

- **GTF chromium** (glucose tolerance factor) has helped many people control sugar cravings. Chromium is an essential trace mineral that helps balance blood sugar and combats insulin resistance. In fact sugar cravings can be a sign of a mineral deficiency for some people. A very large percentage of Americans are low on chromium due to deficiencies in the food they eat, particularly the white flour products. Chromium is needed for insulin to work effectively to transport glucose into your cells for energy. A deficiency in chromium might cause you to have intense sugar cravings. Before supplementing with chromium, however, it's good to consult with your doctor because it should not be taken if you have kidney problems, are allergic to leather, or if you are taking certain medications.

- **L-Glutamine** is very important for digestive health and is especially helpful for the colon. This amino acid heals tissues in the body, especially irritated tissue in the digestive tract. It is known as the calming amino acid and is very effective at reducing anxiety as well as sugar and alcohol cravings. The recommended daily intake is 20 to 25 micrograms for women and 30 to 35 micrograms for men.

- **B vitamins** play a key in insulin metabolism. Your body needs the various B vitamins for insulin to function correctly at different levels of metabolism. You may be deficient if you have eaten white flour products and very little meat, as is the case with many vegetarians.

- **Zinc** is necessary to produce and release insulin. This mineral extends the action of insulin so it does not break down. Many people are zinc-deficient and instead have toxic levels of copper, iron, lead, mercury, or cadmium in their systems—all can replace zinc in the insulin molecule, causing it to malfunction and become very fragile. This fragility can be a major contributor to insulin resistance.

- **Magnesium** is a very important mineral because it affects hundreds of cell interactions throughout the body, such as in the brain, bones, and muscles. It's important for good sleep, normal blood pressure, balanced mood, relief of muscle cramps, restless leg syndrome, charley horses, prevention of constipation, and reduction of powerful chocolate cravings. Roughly 60 percent of the population is estimated to be deficient in magnesium for a variety of reasons. American soil is depleted and no longer rich in magnesium, and many of us don't eat enough foods—especially dark leafy greens, nuts, and beef—that are good sources of magnesium.

- **Vitamin C** can help you detoxify and balance your system. Start with 1,000 mg of pure ascorbic acid (vitamin C) powder or capsules. Work up to what your body needs right now by increasing by 500 mg a day until you reach bowel tolerance. This is the point of a loose stool. Then you cut back by 500 mg at a time until you reach a normal stool. That is the indicator of the amount of vitamin C you need at this time.

9. Sleep well; sleep enough

Getting less sleep or disturbed, fitful sleep causes your appetite hormones to get out of whack. Ghrelin, the appetite-stimulating hormone, shoots up, and leptin, the appetite-control hormone, dives down. A study in the *American Journal of Clinical Nutrition* found that people were more apt to choose high-carb snacks for late-night binges when they were deprived of sleep.[5] According to WebMD, "in a review of 18 studies, researchers found that a lack of sleep led to increased cravings for energy-dense, high-carbohydrate foods."[6]

"During nights of sleep deprivation, you feel that your eating goes wacky," says researcher Robert Stickgold. "Up at 2 a.m., working on a paper, a steak or pasta is not very attractive. You'll grab the candy bar instead. It probably has to do with the glucose regulation going off. It could be that a good chunk of our epidemic of obesity is actually an epidemic of sleep deprivation."[7] When you don't get enough sleep, you want more energy, so you go for quickly absorbed simple carbohydrates for quick energy—sugar. Sleep is an important way to fight against the drive to overeat carbs. You literally can sleep your cravings away. Get seven to nine hours of sleep a night. Determine what your body needs, and don't scrimp.

10. Fight sugar cravings with fat

Fat produces satiety—that feeling of fullness, the feeling that you've had enough to eat. It helps to balance your blood sugar and is necessary for transporting fat soluble vitamins. Choose only good fats—extra-virgin olive oil, coconut oil, avocados, and omega-3 fats from fish and fish oil, seeds, nuts, and nut and seed butters. You need plenty of omega-3 fats for good brain health too.

FIGHT SUGAR CRAVINGS WITH BEANS

One study showed that beans with rice can reduce the glycemic response compared to rice alone, and showed that beans helped the management of type 2 diabetes.[8] Dr. Joel Fuhrman says, "Even though beans are high in protein, it is the special type of carbohydrates in beans that cause these effects....You would never think beans would help you break your sugar addiction, but studies show that people who ate beans at one meal, were able to lessen their glycemic reaction at (a) second meal....This happens because the good bacteria that proliferate in our gut as a result of eating beans produces a certain chemical that slows the rate in which food leaves our stomach and intestines. So those beans are still doing their work at your second meal and even the days that follow if you eat beans regularly, preventing that insulin spike associated with further cravings and fat storage."[9] All beans, including lentils and dried peas, are good. Dr. Fuhrman recommends that you eat at least half a cup of beans every day. Make a big soup on the weekend with plenty of beans, make bean burgers, chili, and stews with beans, and add beans to big salads. Beans are powerful at preventing heart disease and cancer and extending life span—a huge win for your health.[10]

Basic Food Plan

Following is a list of foods to avoid and a list of foods you can eat.

Foods to Avoid

It's time to knock out any opponent to your vibrant health. You're in the ring, in the fight of your life against the bad guys. It's time to deliver the winning punch and claim your healthy new body! Though some of this is a review because I've mentioned it before, it's a good reminder to avoid the items on this list. Avoid these foods for thirty days, and then keep avoiding them as a lifestyle with the exception that you can add in some healthy sweeteners.

Sweeteners

Sugar in all forms: agave nectar, barley malt, agave syrup, pancake syrup, beet sugar, cane sugar, cane juice, confectioner's sugar, organic cane sugar, corn syrup, corn sugar, corn sweetener, corn syrup solids, crystallized fructose, date sugar, dextran, dextrose, high-fructose corn syrup, diastase, diastatic malt, erythritol, evaporated cane juice, fructose, fruit juice concentrate, golden syrup, honey, invert sugar, lactose, malt, maltitol, maltodextrin, maltose, mannitol, maple syrup, glucose, molasses, neotame, polydextrose, raw sugar, refiner's syrup, sorbitol, sorghum syrup, Sucanat, sucrose, stevia, sugar, turbinado sugar, yellow sugar, xylitol, and Zerose.

Artificial sweeteners: sucralose (Splenda), aspartame (Equal or NutraSweet), saccharin (Sweet'N Low).

Beverages

- Coffee, especially with sugar, artificial sweeteners, or sugar-free syrup
- Soda

- Diet soda
- Fruit juice, with the exception of a little low-sugar fruit such as green apple or berries to sweeten vegetable juices or green smoothies
- Sweetened teas
- Energy drinks (regular and diet)
- Dessert wines
- All alcohol

Condiments

- Jam/jelly
- Ketchup
- Salad dressings with any added sugars or sweeteners
- Nut butters with added sugars or sweeteners
- BBQ sauce
- Teriyaki sauce

Meats

All packaged meats, such as turkey, ham, or salami with added sugar

Dairy

Cheese, cream sauces, ice cream, yogurt (except for probiotic plain unsweetened yogurt)—due to milk sugar (lactose)

Desserts (that's *all* desserts)

- Cakes, cookies, pies, doughnuts, and other baked goods
- Candy and chocolate

- Energy bars
- Ice cream, frozen yogurt, Popsicles, and all frozen treats

Miscellaneous

- Cereals
- Breads
- Pasta sauce (with any added sugars or sweeteners)
- Dried fruit
- Energy bars and granola bars (with any added sugars or sweeteners)
- Chewing gum (regular and sugar-free)

Foods You Can Eat

Fruits

Eat fresh or frozen fruit with no sugar added; low-sugar fruits are best, like apples and berries.

Vegetables

You can eat all vegetables, though for the first thirty days it's best to minimize the starchy vegetables and avoid white potatoes as much as possible. If you're craving something sweet, roasting veggies caramelizes their sugars and brings out their sweetness. A baked sweet potato can help as well.

Proteins

Choose clean proteins such as organic, free-range, and grass-fed items. This includes:

- Meat
- Poultry

- Fish (wild-caught only)
- Legumes (beans, peas, lentils)
- Eggs (pastured, organic)
- Tofu (only organic, non-GMO, and in small amounts)
- Nuts (not honey-roasted)
- Seeds

Grains

Choose only whole grains without any added sugars or sweeteners. Avoid flour products. It's best to choose the ancient grains and cook them yourself.

- Brown/wild/red rice
- Quinoa
- Buckwheat
- Millet
- Amaranth
- Teff
- Kamut

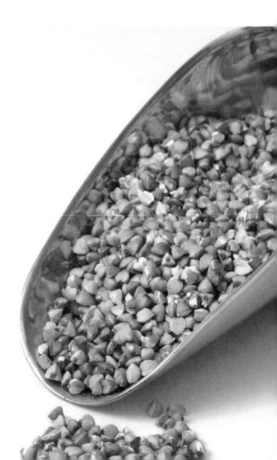

Beverages

- Water
- Seltzer/sparkling water (including naturally flavored, but no added sugar)
- Unsweetened teas (all varieties, including herbal)
- Plant milk, unsweetened: almond milk, cashew milk, coconut milk, or hemp milk
- Pure coconut water

Condiments and Miscellaneous

- All spices and seasonings (choose spices with sweet flavors like cinnamon and nutmeg when you crave sweets)
- Mustard
- All vinegars
- Homemade dressing: make a tasty dressing with apple cider vinegar or balsamic vinegar, Dijon mustard, olive oil, herbs, and sea salt
- Lemon/lime juice and lemon/lime zest
- Salsa (without added sugars or sweeteners)
- Hot sauce (without added sugars or sweeteners)
- Guacamole
- Hummus
- Bragg's liquid aminos or coconut aminos
- Pesto

- Coconut oil, extra-virgin olive oil, and grape seed oil; ghee
- Unsweetened cocoa powder

Sample Menu Plan

Breakfast

Vegetable juice cocktail and/or healthy nut smoothie or green smoothie

And/or scrambled eggs and sautéed vegetables

Green, white, or herbal tea (a squeeze of lemon is nice)

Mid-morning snack

Herbal tea, vegetable juice, or coconut water

Half-dozen sun-dried or naturally processed green or black organic olives or a handful of raw almonds

Lunch

Bean or vegetable soup with salad

1 veggie dehydrated cracker or brown rice cracker

Mid-afternoon snack

Unsweetened herbal iced tea

Handful of sunflower seeds

Dinner

Baked chicken and vegetables

Quinoa

Mixed green salad with your favorite homemade dressing

Dessert

For thirty days you will not eat any sweets to give yourself a complete palate cleanse and a chance to get your sugar cravings under control. You can have low-sugar fruit during this time. Then you can add in desserts and treats made with healthy sweeteners. There are many delicious recipes in the next chapter.

Remember: a sugar-free life is sweet!

Chapter 10

ENJOYING YOUR VICTORY: DESSERTS WITH HEALTHY SWEETENERS

I RARELY MAKE DESSERTS, usually just for special occasions like Thanksgiving and an occasional birthday party. On the following pages I've included my favorite Raw Vegan "Cheesecake" and holiday pumpkin pie that are my standbys. But I also wanted you to have a variety of healthy dessert recipes to choose from. So I asked my friend, vegan chef Vicki Chelf, if she could share some of her delicious healthy dessert recipes for this chapter. I first met Vicki when we collaborated on a book (*Cooking for Life*) that incorporated leftover pulp from juicing into a variety of recipes. Well, things have now come full circle, and Vicki has written a new book entitled *Pulp Kitchen* that has the same theme. She's been generous to share some of her lovely recipes from that book and from *Vicki's Vegan Kitchen*. There are a few of my own recipes from other books here too, along with several new ones. I hope you find some healthy desserts here that you can enjoy. These recipes can be used after your first thirty days of sugar detox.

Raw Vegan "Cheesecake"

From *The Juice Lady's Anti-Inflammation Diet*

3 cups raw cashews, soaked 4 hours to overnight
½ cup fresh lemon juice
¼ cup coconut nectar or pure maple syrup or 1 Tbsp. coconut nectar with ¼ tsp. liquid stevia
½ cup coconut oil, melted
2 tsp. pure vanilla extract
Water as needed

Put soaked cashews, lemon juice, sweetener, coconut oil, and vanilla in a high-speed blender such as Vitamix and process until creamy. Add water as needed; usually around ¼ cup is needed. Add small amounts of water at a time; you don't want it to be too liquid. You can also use a food processor, but it will not be as creamy as when processed in a high-speed blender.

Note: A regular blender will not work.

Pecan Crust:

1 cup flaked unsweetened coconut
1 cup pecan pieces
½ cup coconut or almond flour
2 tsp. ground cinnamon
2 Tbsp. coconut nectar or pure maple syrup
5 Tbsp. coconut oil

Place all dry ingredients in a food processor and pulse until the mixture is crumbly. Add sweetener and coconut oil and pulse several times in short bursts until crumbs are moist and begin to fall from the sides of the bowl. Put crumbs into a pie plate and spread them evenly. Using your fingers, gently press crumbs across the bottom and up the sides of the pie plate. Place in the freezer for at least thirty minutes to set. Then pour in the filling and refrigerate for at least an hour. Serves 6–8.

Almond Butter Balls

Brand-new recipe from Cherie for *The Juice Lady's Sugar Knockout*

16 oz. almond butter (crunchy or creamy)
1 tsp. cinnamon
¼ tsp. stevia or ¼ cup coconut nectar or to taste
2 cups rolled oats or oat flour
1 cup unsweetened shredded coconut flakes or finely chopped nuts

Mix almond butter, cinnamon, and sweetener together in a bowl. Use oats as they are, or blend them until they assume a powder-like texture or use oat flour. Add oats to the nut butter/sweetener mixture and mix until combined, working with hands. Adjust consistency if necessary. Roll batter into small balls. Wet hands often to prevent mixture from sticking to hands. Roll balls in coconut flakes or chopped nuts. Chill and eat! Makes 40 balls.

Notes: This recipe yields a lot, so you can freeze the balls and grab a few when you need a snack or are craving something sweet. It's worthwhile to make them all at once and freeze them or keep them in the fridge for up to ten days.

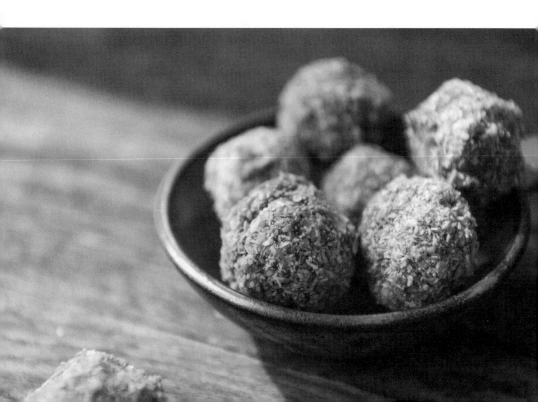

Coconut Pineapple Sorbet

From *The Coconut Diet*

This impressive dessert is so delicious it is hard to believe that it does not contain sugar. To make it you will need a blender, a juicer, and an ice cream maker.

1 cup coconut milk
1 fresh pineapple, peeled and cut into spears
¼ tsp. stevia or other healthy sweetener, to taste
1 tsp. pure vanilla extract
2 Tbsp. virgin coconut oil

Place coconut milk in a large measuring cup. Run pineapple through juicer. Reserve all of the juice and ⅓ cup of the pulp. Place enough of the pineapple juice in the cup with the coconut milk to make 3 cups liquid. If you do not have enough, add a little filtered water. Place liquid mixture in a blender with the remaining ingredients, except for the pulp, and blend. Pour mixture into an ice cream maker, add pulp, and process according to directions until frozen. Enjoy! Serves 6.

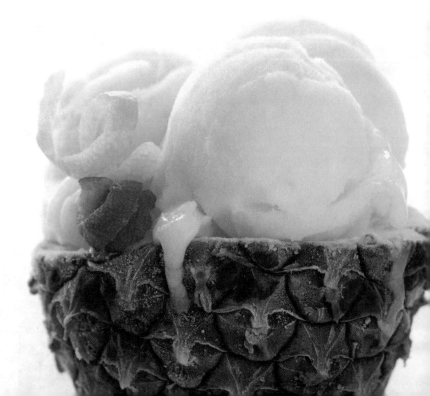

Lemon Torte

From *The Juice Lady's Living Foods Revolution*

Filling:

1 cup cashews, soaked 8 hours
2 lemons, zested
Juice of 2 lemons
2 Tbsp. pure maple syrup
1 orange, juiced
1 Tbsp. psyllium powder

Blend all ingredients except psyllium in a blender until it is the consistency of whipped cream. Fold in psyllium. Pour into tart shell (shortbread crust) and freeze. Take out one hour before serving and refrigerate.

Shortbread Crust:

2 ½ cups shredded unsweetened coconut
½ cup cashews, soaked 1 hour
2 Tbsp. honey or coconut nectar

Put coconut in blender and start on low speed, then high. As a well forms, slowly add cashews to crumbly stage. Then add honey. Use spatula if needed to blend. Blend until mixture heats a little bit.

Press crust in bottom and sides of one large or four small tart pans. Pour in lemon filling. Cover with plastic wrap, and freeze for at least one hour. Take out and put in refrigerator thirty minutes before serving. Serves 4.

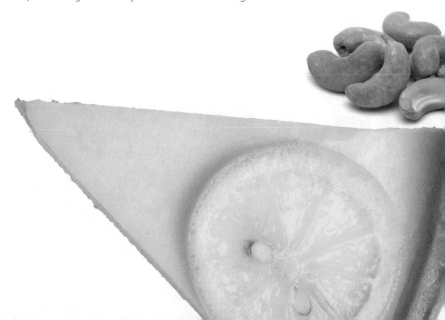

Summer Peach Parfait

From *The Juice Lady's Living Foods Revolution*

2 cups raw almonds
7 peaches
4 Tbsp. raw almond butter
¼ cup coconut nectar
¼ cup fresh orange juice
2 Tbsp. vanilla
2 tsp. cinnamon
4 tsp. nutmeg
Pinch Celtic sea salt
2 pints of blueberries (optional)

Soak almonds in 3 cups of purified water for six to twelve hours. Peel and thinly slice the peaches. In a blender blend 1 peeled peach and remaining ingredients except blueberries. Add more orange juice as needed to aid in blending until a custard consistency is reached. In parfait glasses, layer peaches, custard, peaches, custard, and top with blueberries. Serves 6.

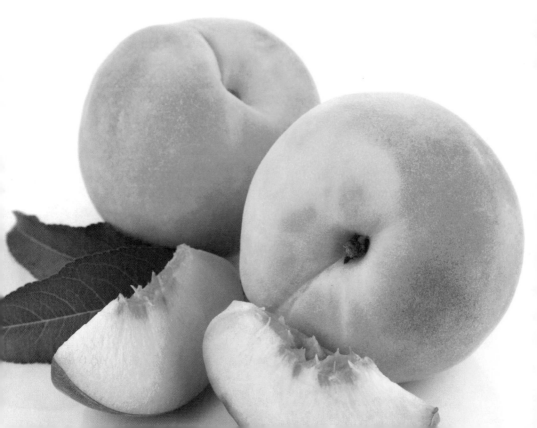

Gluten-Free, Sugar-Free Carrot Cake

Brand new recipe from Cherie for *The Juice Lady's Sugar Knockout*

For your next birthday party or special event, here's a cake that is both delicious and healthful.

Cake

Dry Ingredients:

½ cup ground pumpkin seeds
¼ cup coconut flour
1 tsp. baking powder
1 tsp. cinnamon
½ tsp. allspice

Wet Ingredients:

4 pastured organic eggs
2 cups shredded carrots (you can use leftover carrot pulp from juicing)
¼ cup unsweetened applesauce
½ cup sunflower seed butter
½ cup coconut nectar

Preheat oven to 325 degrees. Add unbleached parchment paper to the bottom of two 8-inch round greased cake pans. Combine all of the dry ingredients. Whisk the eggs until frothy in a small bowl. Combine carrots, applesauce, and sunflower seed butter in a large bowl. Stir in eggs and combine. Add dry ingredients to the wet ingredients, and stir until well combined. Divide the batter between the two cake pans and bake for 25–30 minutes or until a toothpick comes out clean.

Dairy-Free "Cream Cheese" Frosting

1 cup coconut oil
1 cup coconut yogurt, unsweetened
1 cup cream off the top of a can of full-fat coconut milk (get coconut milk without additives/emulsifiers like guar gum; you want only the cream off the top)
1 tsp. pure vanilla extract
3 Tbsp. coconut nectar

Put all ingredients in a blender and process until smooth. Allow the mixture to set in the refrigerator for several hours or overnight. When icing has set, divide in two parts and spread a layer on the top of each cake layer. Chill and serve. Serves 8.

Note: If you are not sensitive to dairy, you can use a cream cheese frosting made with a healthy sweetener.

Gluten-Free Sugar-Free Dairy-Free Pumpkin Pie

Brand new recipe from Cherie for *The Juice Lady's Sugar Knockout*

Crust:

1 cup almonds or pecans, finely ground in blender until flour-like, or almond flour
3 Tbsp. coconut oil plus some extra to grease pie pan
1 free-range organic egg
½ tsp. cinnamon powder

Preheat oven to 325 degrees. Grease pie pan with coconut oil and mix crust ingredients by hand in a medium-sized bowl. Press crust into bottom and sides of pie pan and put in the oven while making the filling. Remove the crust as it barely starts to brown (10 to 15 minutes).

Filling:

1 (15-oz.) can of unsweetened pumpkin, or about 2 cups homemade pureed pumpkin (drain excess liquid)
3 free-range organic eggs
¼ cup pure maple syrup + ⅛ tsp. stevia
1 Tbsp. pumpkin pie spice
1 tsp. pure vanilla extract
1 (13.5-oz.) can of full-fat coconut milk

In medium bowl, combine filling ingredients and mix using a food processor or Vitamix. A hand mixer will not get it as smooth! It should be smooth and spreadable, but not pourable. Spread the filling over the crust and return to oven for about an hour or until center is firm and a toothpick comes out clean. It will set more as it cooks.

Coconut Whipped Cream:

½ cup full-fat coconut milk, chilled (get coconut milk without emulsifiers such as guar gum; use only the cream on the top)
½ tsp. pure vanilla extract
1 tsp. coconut nectar, or a few drops of stevia

For the coconut whipped cream, combine all ingredients listed in a medium bowl that has been chilled. Using a hand mixer, whip at high speed for a minute or two until it becomes fluffy and peaks like whipped cream. Chill until ready to serve.

Top the pie with coconut whipped cream. Serves 6–8.

Blueberry Crumble

From *Vicki's Vegan Kitchen* by Vicki Chelf

This is a recipe that everyone loves. It is best with fresh berries but will still be very good with frozen. By using both stevia and a bit of coconut sugar, it is almost impossible to tell that there is stevia in the recipe.

1 cup rolled oats
1 cup walnuts
¼ cup coconut oil
2 Tbsp. coconut sugar
1 tsp. vanilla
1 tsp. liquid stevia
4 cups blueberries

Place rolled oats, walnuts, coconut oil, coconut sugar, vanilla, and stevia in a food processor. Blend until nuts are ground and ingredients are combined. Wash blueberries, picking out any stems or damaged berries, and place them in the bottom of an 8" by 8" oven dish. Spread flour mixture over berries. Bake at 350 degrees for 30 minutes or until the berries are bubbly and the top is brown. Serves 6.

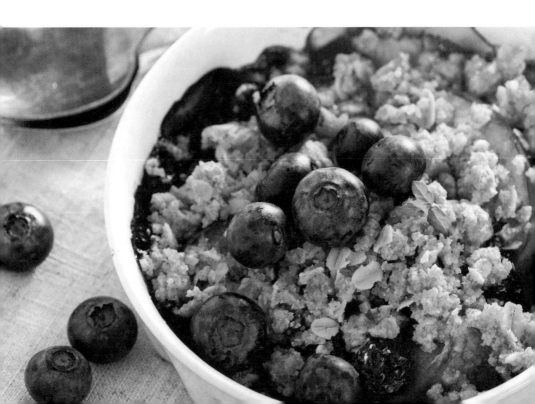

Apple Crisp

From *Vicki's Vegan Kitchen* by Vicki Chelf

This wholesome, wheatless, easy-to-make dessert is delicious served plain, either warm or cold. It is also good hot from the oven, topped with vegan ice cream.

Apple Mixture:

6 medium apples, sliced (2½ to 2¾ pounds)
2 Tbsp. lemon juice
2 Tbsp. coconut syrup

Place sliced apples in a shallow baking dish. Sprinkle them with lemon juice and then drizzle coconut syrup over them.

Topping:

2 cups rolled oats
⅓ cup unrefined coconut oil
1 tsp. vanilla
2 tsp. cinnamon
½ tsp. cardamom
⅓ cup coconut syrup

Place oats and oil in a food processor. Blend until well-combined. Keep blending and add vanilla, cinnamon, and cardamom. Continue blending and drizzle in coconut syrup. Blend for a few seconds more to mix the dough.

Distribute this mixture over the top of the apple mixture. Use a wet fork to spread it out and flatten it out somewhat. Don't worry if it looks a little sloppy. It will look just fine after it bakes.

Bake at 350 degrees for 50 minutes, or until fruit is tender and bubbly and the top is crispy brown. Serves 6.

Variations:

- Substitute ½ cup raisins or currants for the coconut syrup that is added to the apples and add about ¼ cup apple juice or water to the pan with the fruit.

- Substitute pears, blueberries, or blackberries for part of the apples.

- Add about ½ cup chopped walnuts or pecans to the topping.

Fruit and Nut Squares

From *Vicki's Vegan Kitchen* by Vicki Chelf

This recipe is a longtime favorite. You can vary the types of dried fruits, juices, sweeteners, and flours, and it always works.

2 cups date pieces, or pitted cooking dates
1 cup raisins
2 tsp. vanilla
1¼ cup peach nectar or other fruit juice
2 cups walnuts
1 cup oat or sorghum flour
¼ cup coconut sugar
1 tsp. cinnamon
¼ cup coconut oil

Place date pieces, raisins, vanilla, and fruit juice in a saucepan. Bring to a boil. Cover, reduce the heat, and simmer for about 5 minutes or until the liquid has been absorbed and dates have formed a puree. Set aside.

Place 1 cup of walnuts in a blender or food processor and grind them. Place remaining nuts on a cutting board and coarsely chop them with a sharp knife. Place all nuts in a mixing bowl. Add flour, coconut sugar, and cinnamon. Mix well. With a fork, slowly stir in oil and mix until oil is thoroughly incorporated into the mixture. The mixture should look like coarse crumbs.

Sprinkle a little more than half of the crumb mixture evenly into a lightly oiled 8" by 8" baking dish. Spread the date puree evenly over the crumb mixture, and sprinkle the surface with the remaining crumb mixture. Lightly press the crumb mixture into the date puree.

Bake at 350 degrees for 25 minutes. Cut into 2-inch squares. Let cool for about 30 minutes before removing from the pan. Makes about 32 2-inch squares.

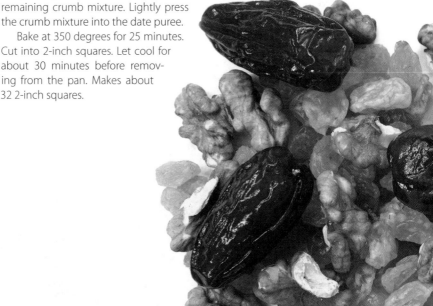

Chocolate Macadamia Nut Mousse

From *Vicki's Vegan Kitchen* by Vicki Chelf

This recipe is so simple that even people who think that they can't make desserts will be amazed at how easy it is.

½ cup macadamia nuts
½ cup plant milk
¼ cup coconut sugar
¼ cup cocoa powder
2 tsp. pure vanilla
Shaved dark chocolate and/or chopped macadamia nuts, for garnish

Place macadamia nuts and plant milk in a blender and blend until very smooth and creamy. Add sugar, cocoa powder, and vanilla and blend again, using a rubber spatula to scrape the sides of the blender if necessary. Serve in pretty little stemmed glasses and sprinkle with chopped macadamia nuts or shaved chocolate. This pudding is also good as a topping for a plain cake.

Avocado Mousse

From *Vicki's Vegan Kitchen* by Vicki Chelf

This recipe is not the usual use for avocados, but it is scrumptious and very pretty. For an exotic touch, substitute goji berries for the strawberries or raspberries.

1 Florida avocado or 2 California avocados
¼ cup coconut syrup, or to taste
1 tsp. vanilla extract
2 Tbsp. lemon juice
½-inch piece lemon peel
Approximately ¼ cup almond milk, as needed
Fresh strawberries or raspberries
Finely grated coconut

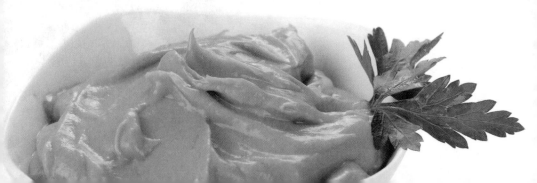

Cut avocado or avocados in half lengthwise. Remove pit and scoop out flesh. Place flesh in a blender along with coconut syrup, vanilla, lemon juice, and lemon peel. Blend until smooth and creamy, adding as much milk as needed to make it blendable. Taste and add more sweetener if necessary.

Put the mousse in chilled sherbet glasses. Top with strawberries or raspberries and sprinkle with a little grated coconut. Chill until ready to serve. Serves 4–6.

Variation:

Chocolate Mousse: This mousse can be turned into a chocolate one by omitting the lemon and adding about ¼ cup cocoa powder, to taste. If the mousse gets too thick, add a bit of extra plant milk. Adjust sweetener to taste.

Chocolate Peanut Pulp Balls

From *Pulp Kitchen* by Vicki Chelf

I was truly amazed at how good these are, and no one would know they contain pulp unless you tell them! In a Vitamix blender, they are really easy to make. A food processor will work, but you will have to work a little harder to get the mixture ground up.

1 cup carrot pulp
1 cup soft medjool dates (about 14)
½ cup cocoa powder
¾ cup crunchy peanut butter
½ cup dry unsweetened shredded coconut or ground peanuts

Place pulp in a large bowl.

Place dates, cocoa powder, and peanut butter in a Vitamix blender or food processor. An ordinary blender will not work. Blend until relatively smooth using the Vitamix plunger to help you along. In a food processor you will have to stop the machine occasionally and scrape the sides with a rubber spatula to get it blended properly.

Add blended mixture to the bowl with the pulp and knead it together, using your hands. Roll the mixture into balls, slightly smaller than walnuts.

Place unsweetened coconut or ground peanuts in a small bowl. Roll the balls in the coconut or peanut mixture. Store in the refrigerator or freezer. Makes approximately 26 balls.

Variation:

Substitute almond butter with ½ teaspoon of almond extract for the peanut butter, and roll the balls in ground almonds, either raw or toasted.

Stuffed Figs

From *Vicki's Vegan Kitchen* by Vicki Chelf

Here's an exotic dessert that is perfect for an afternoon buffet, a gourmet treat, or even to carry in your backpack on a ski or hiking trip.

18–20 large brown dried figs
Water or apple juice to cover (optional)
1 cup ground pecans
¼ cup finely shredded unsweetened coconut
½ tsp. cardamom
18–20 pecan halves

If the figs are soft and fresh, they may be stuffed without soaking. However, if they are hard, soak them overnight, or until soft, in water or apple juice to cover. Cut the stem end off of the figs. Using your fingers, open up each fig to form a pouch. Mix together ground pecans, coconut, and cardamom. Stuff figs with nut mixture and top each with a pecan half. Makes approximately 18–20 stuffed figs.

Note: If figs have to be soaked, this dessert must be stored in the refrigerator.

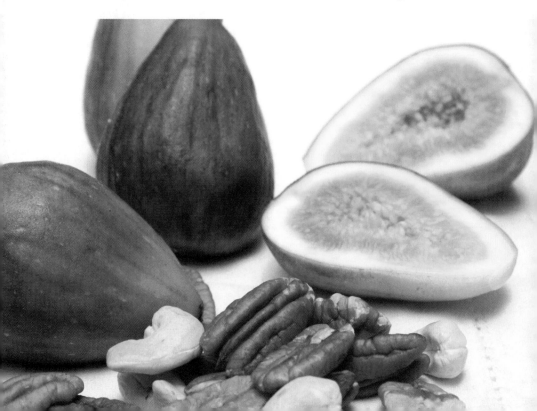

Beet Brownies

From *Pulp Kitchen* by Vicki Chef

Here is a really good gluten-free brownie that hides a good dose of beet pulp within its dark chocolate deliciousness. I find most brownie recipes unpleasantly sweet, so I created one that I thought was scrumptious without being cloying. All the ingredients have ½ cup measure, except for the vanilla and baking powder, so it should be easy to make!

½ cup mashed organic silken tofu (medium firmness)
½ cup beet juice, vegan milk, or water
½ cup maple syrup or coconut syrup
½ cup coconut oil
1 tsp. vanilla
½ cup garbanzo flour
½ cup cocoa powder
1½ tsp. baking powder
½ cup beet pulp
½ cup vegan chocolate chips
½ cup chopped nuts, or cacao nibs

Combine tofu, beet juice (or other liquid), maple syrup, coconut oil, and vanilla in a blender and blend until smooth and creamy. In a mixing bowl sift together flour, cocoa, and baking powder. Mix well. Add pulp, and mix to distribute it evenly throughout the flour. Then stir in chocolate chips and nuts. Add blended mixture to flour mixture. Mix well to combine ingredients and form a batter.

Transfer the batter into an 8" by 8" baking pan that has been generously oiled and floured. Bake at 350 degrees for about 25 minutes or until firm to the touch. Let cool in pan before slicing and removing.

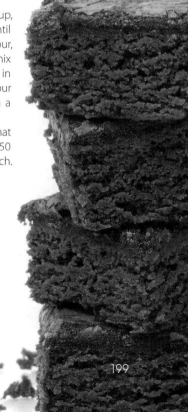

Carrot Date Squares, or Carrot Halwa

From *Pulp Kitchen* by Vicki Chef

This is an easy way to turn carrot pulp into a delectable treat. And you have two choices: either serve it as a pudding-style dish or as candy squares.

1 cup carrot pulp (6–8 carrots)
½ cup soft pitted dates
½ cup almonds
½ cup cashews
1 tsp. coconut butter
½ tsp. cardamom
2 Tbsp. chopped pistachios or unsweetened shredded coconut

Place all ingredients, except for pistachios or coconut, in a food processor and grind until sticky enough to hold together. If you like, you can stop here and transfer the mixture to 8 small dessert cups and garnish with pistachios. This will taste a lot like the Indian sweet carrot halwa, but it is a lot more nutritious. If you wish to make squares, continue to the next step.

Sprinkle half of coconut in the bottom of a 5" by 8½" loaf pan. Place the mixture in the pan to cover the bottom in a somewhat even layer. Press firmly so the mixture holds together. Sprinkle remaining coconut over the top and press it in. Cut it into 8 approximately 1¾-inch squares. Store in a covered container in the refrigerator.

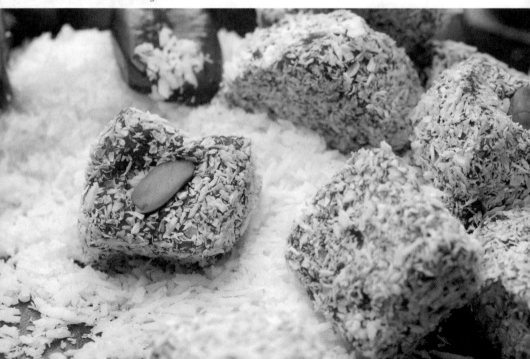

Coconut Cookies

From *Pulp Kitchen* by Vicki Chelf

These cookies are very high in protein, partly sweetened with stevia, gluten-free, and high in fiber.

1 cup chickpea flour
2 tsp. baking powder
¼ tsp. baking soda
1 cup carrot pulp
1 cup shredded unsweetened coconut
⅓ cup coconut butter
⅓ cup coconut nectar or maple syrup
½ dropper-full liquid stevia, or to taste
2 tsp. vanilla

In a large bowl, combine chickpea flour, baking powder, and baking soda. Mix well. Add pulp and coconut. Mix well, and rub the mixture together in your hands to distribute the pulp fairly evenly throughout the mixture.

In a separate bowl, combine coconut butter, coconut nectar or maple syrup, stevia, and vanilla. Mix well.

Add sweet mixture to flour mixture, and knead with your hands to form a dough. Roll dough out onto the counter to make a thick log that is about 10 inches long. Cut the log into about twenty ¼-inch-thick pieces using a sharp, thin knife that has been dipped in cool water. Place the pieces on an oiled cookie sheet. At this point you can use your hands to reshape them a bit, then flatten them slightly with the tines of a fork dipped in cool water.

Bake at 350 degrees for 15–20 minutes or until firm and lightly browned on the bottom. They should be a bit like shortbread. They can be eaten warm out of the oven, or if you want them to be crispier, you can turn off the oven, but leave them in until the oven is cool so they dry out a bit. Makes approximately 20 cookies.

Papaya Pie

From *Pulp Kitchen* by Vicki Chelf

This pie is totally raw with a fabulously creamy texture that holds up for slicing. It is easy to make. Crust:

1 cup almonds
½ cup soft pitted dates
¼ tsp. salt

Place almonds, dates, and salt in a food processor and process until the mixture is finely ground. Press mixture into a 9-inch pie pan.

Filling:

1 medium papaya (about 2 to 2½ pounds)
½ cup soft pitted dates
¼ cup coconut butter

Peel and seed papaya. Cut into strips and juice. Reserve 2 cups juice and all the pulp. Place juice in a blender or food processor with dates and coconut butter. Blend until very smooth and creamy. Transfer the mixture to a bowl and add pulp. Mix well and pour into piecrust. Refrigerate for at least 3 hours before slicing.

Banana Pecan Ice Cream

Created by Vicki Chef

You need a Vitamix or other high-power blender for this recipe. The pecans turn the frozen bananas into an amazingly rich and delicious treat!

4 peeled and frozen bananas
⅓ cup pecans
1–4 Tbsp. vegan milk, as needed

Place bananas in Vitamix and blend, adding a little milk if needed to make it blend smooth. Add pecans and blend again, but do not blend until it is totally smooth; leave some small pieces in the ice cream. Scrape out the mixture as quickly as possible and serve immediately, topped with extra pecans, if desired. Serves 4–6.

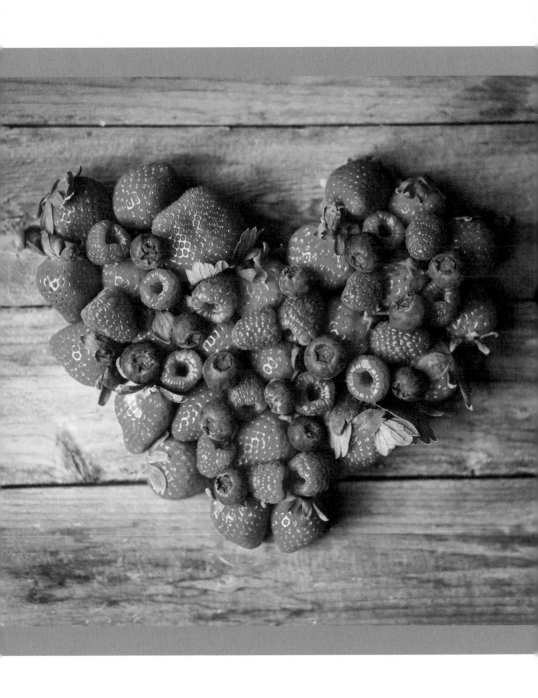

Appendix

RESOURCES

S IGN UP FOR the Juice Lady's free Juicy Tips Newsletter at www.juiceladyinfo.com.

Cherie's Websites

- www.juiceladyinfo.com, www.juiceladycherie.com, or www.cheriecalbom.com—information on juicing and weight loss
- www.gococonuts.com—information about the Coconut Diet and coconut oil

The Juice Lady's Health and Wellness Juice Cleanse Retreats

I invite you to join us for a week that can change your life! Our retreats offer gourmet organic raw foods with a three-day juice fast midweek. We present interesting, informative classes in a beautiful, peaceful setting where you can experience healing and restoration of body and soul. For more information and dates for the retreats, visit http://www.juiceladycherie.com/Juice/juice-raw-food-retreat/ or call 866-843-8935.

The Juice Lady's Jumpstart Health and Fitness 8-Week E-Course

The eight-week e-course helps you achieve your health and fitness goals. I lead you step-by-step to better health and fitness. I want you to embrace your own healthy lifestyle that you can stick with for life. For more information, go to http://www.juiceladycherie.com/Juice /healthy-and-fit-for-life/ or call 866-843-8935.

The Juice Lady's 30-Day Detox Challenge

This is a 4-week e-course designed to help your body get rid of toxins, contaminants, waste, and heavy metals that can accumulate in joints, organs, tissues, cells, the lymphatic system, and the bloodstream. It can energize your entire body. For more information, go to http://www.juiceladycherie.com/Juice/30-day-detox/ or call 866-843-8935.

Healthy Holiday Cooking, Juicing, and Entertaining in Style 4-week E-Course

This class is designed to help you navigate through the holiday season with health choices and keep your waistline. Weekly you'll get recipes and health tips plus ideas to overcome emotional eating. Enjoy "Yummy Juices, Treats, Appetizers, and Main Dishes."

Nutrition Consultation

To schedule a nutrition consultation with the Juice Lady's team, visit http://www.juiceladycherie.com/Juice/nutritional-counseling/ or call 866-843-8935.

Scheduling Cherie Calbom to Speak

To schedule Cherie Calbom to speak for your organization, call 866-843-8935.

Books by Cherie and John Calbom

These books can be ordered at any of the websites above or by calling 866-8GETWEL (866-843-8935).

- Cherie Calbom, Abby Fammartino, *The Juice Lady's Anti-Inflammation Diet* (Siloam Press).
- Cherie Calbom, *The Juice Lady's Big Book of Juices and Green Smoothies* (Siloam Press).
- Cherie Calbom, *The Juice Lady's Remedies for Asthma and Allergies* (Siloam Press).
- Cherie Calbom, *The Juice Lady's Remedies for Stress and Adrenal Fatigue* (Siloam Press).
- Cherie Calbom, *The Juice Lady's Weekend Weight-Loss Diet* (Siloam Press).
- Cherie Calbom, *The Juice Lady's Living Foods Revolution* (Siloam Press).
- Cherie Calbom, *The Juice Lady's Turbo Diet* (Siloam Press).
- Cherie Calbom, *The Juice Lady's Guide to Juicing for Health* (Avery).
- Cherie Calbom and John Calbom, *Juicing, Fasting, and Detoxing for Life* (Wellness Central).
- Cherie Calbom, *The Wrinkle Cleanse* (Avery).
- Cherie Calbom and John Calbom, *The Coconut Diet* (Wellness Central).
- Cherie Calbom, John Calbom, and Michael Mahaffey, *The Complete Cancer Cleanse* (Thomas Nelson).
- Cherie Calbom, *The Ultimate Smoothie Book* (Wellness Central).

Juicers

To find out about the best juicers recommended by Cherie, call 866-8GETWEL (866-843-8935) or visit www.juiceladyinfo.com.

Dehydrators

To find out the best dehydrators recommended by Cherie, call 866-8GETWEL (866-843-8935) or visit www.juiceladyinfo.com.

Lymphasizer

To view the Swing Machine (lymphasizer), visit www.juicelady-info.com or call 866-8GETWEL (866-843-8935).

Veggie Powders and Supplements

To purchase or get information on Wheatgrass Juice Powder, Barley Max, Carrot Juice Max, and Beet Max powders, go to www. juiceladyinfo.com or call 866-8GETWEL (866-843-8935). (These powders are ideal for when you travel or when you can't get juice.)

Internal Cleansing Kits

The complete and comprehensive internal cleansing kit contains eighteen items for a twenty-one-day cleanse program. You will receive a free colon cleanse kit, along with Liver-Gallbladder Rejuvenator, Friendly Bacteria Replenisher, Parasite Cleanser, Lung Rejuvenator, Kidney and Bladder Rejuvenator, Blood and Skin Rejuvenator, and Lymph Rejuvenator. See website for more information. You may order the cleansing products and get the 10 percent discount by calling 866-843-8935.

Berry Breeze

Keep your produce fresher longer and your fridge smelling fresh too. It can save you up to $2,200 a year from lost produce. Go to www.juiceladycherie.com.

NOTES

Introduction
It's Time to Knock Out That Sweet Tooth!

1. Nicole M. Avena, Pedro Rada, and Bartley G. Hoebel, "Evidence for Sugar Addiction: Behavioral and Neurochemical Effects of Intermittent, Excessive Sugar Intake," *Neuroscience and Biobehavioral Reviews* 32, no. 1 (2008): 20–39. doi:10.1016/j.neubiorev .2007.04.019.

2. Carlo Colantuoni et al., "Evidence That Intermittent, Excessive Sugar Intake Causes Endogenous Opioid Dependence," *Obesity Research* 10, no. 6 (June 2002), 478–488. doi:10.1038/oby.2002.66.

Chapter 1
Sugar's Low Blow to Our Health and Wellness

1. Gary Taubes, "Is Sugar Toxic?" *New York Times*, April 13, 2011, accessed July 12, 2015, http://www.nytimes .com/2011/04/17/magazine/mag-17Sugar-t.html?_r=0.

2. Ibid.

3. Ibid.

4. Ibid.

5. Cynthia L. Ogden et al., "Prevalence of Obesity in the United States, 2009–2010," Centers for Disease Control

and Prevention NCHS Data Brief no. 82, January 2012, http://www.cdc.gov/nchs/data/databriefs/db82.htm; see also "Childhood Obesity Facts," Centers for Disease Control and Prevention, June 19, 2015, http://www.cdc.gov/obesity/data/childhood.html.

6. "National Diabetes Statistics Report: Estimates of Diabetes and Its Burden in the United States, 2014," Centers for Disease Control and Prevention, 2014, http://www.cdc.gov/diabetes/pubs/statsreport14/national-diabetes-report-web.pdf.

7. Dennis Kasper et al., "Harrison's Principles of Internal Medicine, 19e," accessed July 12, 2015, http://accessmedicine.mhmedical.com/book.aspx?bookid=1130.

8. Taubes, "Is Sugar Toxic?"

9. Peter Attia, "Is Sugar Toxic?" *The Eating Academy Blog*, accessed July 10, 2015, http://eatingacademy.com/nutrition/is-sugar-toxic.

10. K. L. Stanhope, J. M. Schwarz, and P. J. Havel, "Adverse Metabolic Effects of Dietary Fructose: Results from the Recent Epidemiological, Clinical, and Mechanistic Studies," *Current Opinion in Lipidology* 24, no. 3 (June 2013): 198–206. doi:10.1097/MOL.0b013e3283613bca.

11. A. Rodgers, "Effect of Cola Consumption on Urinary Biochemical and Physicochemical Risk Factors Associated with Calcium Oxalate Urolithiasis," *Urological Research* 27, no. 1 (1999): 77–81.

12. Joseph Mercola, "Six Ways to Keep Kidney Stones at Bay," Mercola.com, September 29, 2011, accessed July 12, 2015, http://articles.mercola.com/sites/articles /archive/2011/09/29/six-ways-to-keep-kidney-stones -at-bay-from-the-harvard-health-letter.aspx.

13. Harvard Heart Letter, "Abundance of Fructose Not Good for the Liver, Heart," Harvard Health Publications, September 1, 2011, http://www.health.harvard .edu/heart-health/abundance-of-fructose-not-good-for-the- liver-heart.

14. K. M. Utzschneider, S. E. Kahn, "Review: The Role of Insulin Resistance in Nonalcoholic Fatty Liver Disease," *The Journal of Clinical Endocrinology & Metabolism* 91, no. 12 (December 2006): 4753–61.

15. Harvard Heart Letter, "Abundance of Fructose not Good for the Liver, Heart."

16. Ibid.

17. M. E. Bocarsly et al., "High-Fructose Corn Syrup Causes Characteristics of Obesity in Rats: Increased Body Weight, Body Fat and Triglyceride Levels," *Pharmacology, Biochemistry, and Behavior* 97, no. 1 (November 2010): 101–6. doi:10.1016/j.pbb .2010.02.012.

18. Giovanni Targher, Christopher P. Day, and Enzo Bonora, "Risk of Cardiovascular Disease in Patients with Nonalcoholic Fatty Liver Disease," *New England Journal of Medicine* 363 (September 30, 2010): 1341–1350. doi:10.1056/NEJMra0912063.

19. Victor, February 18, 2010, comment on "Corn Syrup Is Fine in Moderation?" Benefits of Honey, accessed July 11, 2015, http://www.benefits-of-honey.com/corn-syrup.html.

20. Joseph Mercola, "Confirmed—Fructose Can Increase Your Hunger and Lead to Overeating," Mercola.com, January 14, 2013, accessed July 12, 2015, http://articles.mercola.com/sites/articles/archive/2013/01/14/fructose-spurs-overeating.aspx.

21. L. J. Durling, L. Busk, and B. E. Hellman, "Evaluation of the DNA Damaging Effect of the Heat-Induced Food Toxicant 5-Hydroxymethylfurfural (HMF) in Various Cell Lines with Different Activities of Sulfotransferases," *Food and Chemical Toxicology* 47, no. 4 (April 2009): 880–4. doi:10.1016/j.fct.2009.01.022.

22. American Chemical Society, "Soda Warning? High-Fructose Corn Syrup Linked to Diabetes, New Study Suggests," Science Daily, August 23, 2007, accessed July 11, 2015, http://www.sciencedaily.com/releases/2007/08/070823094819.htm.

23. Harvard Heart Letter, "Abundance of Fructose not Good for the Liver, Heart."

24. Lisa Parker and Robin Green, "Why Doesn't Baby Formula List Sugar Content?" NBC Chicago, February 14, 2012, accessed July 11, 2015, http://www.nbcchicago.com/investigations/target-5-sugar-baby-formula-139339308.html.

25. Joseph Mercola, "Fructose: This Addictive Commonly Used Food Feeds Cancer Cells, Triggers Weight Gain,

and Promotes Premature Aging," Mercola.com, April 20, 2010, accessed July 11, 2015, http://articles.mercola.com/sites/articles/archive/2010/04/20/sugar-dangers.aspx.

26. William Dufty, "Refined Sugar: The Sweetest Poison of All," EMR Labs, LLC, accessed July 13, 2015, https://www.quantumbalancing.com/news/sugar_blues.htm, extracted/edited from William Dufty, *Sugar Blues* (Padnor, PA: Chilton Book Co., 1975).

27. Carolyn Gregoire, "This Is What Sugar Does to Your Brain," *The Huffington Post*, April 6, 2015, accessed August 26, 2015, http://www.huffingtonpost.com/2015/04/06/sugar-brain-mental-health_n_6904778.html.

28. Ibid.

29. Ibid.

30. Ibid.

31. Ibid.

Chapter 2
Sweet Tooth or Addiction?

1. Kyle S. Burger and Eric Stice, "Frequent Ice Cream Consumption Is Associated with Reduced Striatal Response to Receipt of an Ice Cream–Based Milkshake," *American Journal of Clinical Nutrition* 95, no. 4 (April 2012): 810–817, http://ajcn.nutrition.org/content/95/4/810.long; see also Andrew Hough, "Ice Cream As 'Addictive As Drugs' Says New Study," *The*

Telegraph, March 5, 2012, accessed July 10, 2015, http://www.telegraph.co.uk/news/science/science-news/9118768/Ice-cream-as-addictive-as-drugs-says-new-study.html.

2. Hough, "Ice Cream As 'Addictive As Drugs.'"

3. "Definition of Addiction," American Society of Addiction Medicine, April 19, 2011, accessed July 12, 2015, http://www.asam.org/for-the-public/definition-of-addiction.

4. Ibid.

5. David Benton, "The Plausibility of Sugar Addiction and Its Role in Obesity and Eating Disorders," *Clinical Nutrition* 29, no. 3 (2009): 288–303. doi:http://dx.doi.org/10.1016/j.clnu.2009.12.001, as referenced in Sugar Free Alex, "The Psychology Behind Sugar Addictions," SpoonfulofSugarFree.com, May 28, 2013, accessed September 16, 2015, http://www.spoonfulofsugarfree.com/2013/05/28/the-psychology-behind-sugar-addictions.

6. Belinda S. Lennerz et al., "Effects of Dietary Glycemic Index on Brain Regions Related to Reward and Craving in Men," *American Journal of Clinical Nutrition* (June 26, 2013). doi: 10.3945/ajcn.113.064113, as referenced in Mark Hyman, "5 Clues You Are Addicted to Sugar," November 21, 2014, accessed July 14, 2015, http://drhyman.com/blog/2013/06/27/5-clues-you-are-addicted-to-sugar/.

7. Hyman, "5 Clues You Are Addicted to Sugar."

8. Jacob Sullum, "Research Shows Cocaine and Heroin Are Less Addictive Than Oreos," *Forbes*, October 16, 2013, http://www.forbes.com/sites/jacob-sullum/2013/10/16/research-shows-cocaine-and-heroin-are-less-addictive-than-oreos/.

9. Robin Young and Jeremy Hobson, "Is Sugar More Addictive Than Cocaine?" Here and Now, January 7, 2015, http://hereandnow.wbur.org/2015/01/07/sugar-health-research.

10. S. H. Ahmed, K. Guillem, Y. Vandaele, "Sugar Addiction: Pushing the Drug-Sugar Analogy to the Limit," *Current Opinion in Clinical Nutrition and Metabolic Care* 16, no. 4 (July 2013): 434–9. doi:10.1097/MCO.0b013e328361c8b8.

11. Ibid.

12. Jonathan Benson, "Studies Determine Sugar, Saccharin More Addictive Than Cocaine," Natural News, November 3, 2014, accessed July 14, 2015, http://www.naturalnews.com/047495_sugar_saccharin_addiction.html.

13. Dufty, *Sugar Blues*.

14. Benson, "Studies Determine Sugar, Saccharin More Addictive Than Cocaine."

15. Young and Hobson, "Is Sugar More Addictive Than Cocaine?"

16. Lennerz et al., "Effects of Dietary Glycemic Index," as referenced in Hyman, "5 Clues You Are Addicted to Sugar."

17. Holly Carling, "The Drug No One Wants to Talk About," CDAPress.com, June 26, 2013, http://www.cdapress. com/news/healthy_community/article_e1a51e78-1411-5867-b973-78ff3f696ec5.html.

18. Michael Moss, "The Extraordinary Science of Addictive Junk Food," *New York Times*, February 20, 2013, accessed July 28, 2015, http://www.nytimes. com/2013/02/24/magazine/the-extraordinary-science-of-junk-food.html?_r=0; see also Joseph Mercola, "Sugar Industry Secrets Exposed," Mercola.com, July 25, 2015, accessed July 28, 2015, http://articles.mercola. com/sites/articles/archive/2015/07/25/sugar-industry-secrets.aspx.

19. Mercola, "Sugar Industry Secrets Exposed."

20. Mandy Oaklander, "10 Hidden Sugar Bombs," Prevention, accessed July 28, 2015, http://prevenlion.com/ food/healthy-eating-tips/10-hidden-sugar-bombs.html.

21. Gary Taubes and Cristin Kearns Couzens, "Big Sugar's Sweet Little Lies," *Mother Jones* November/December 2012, accessed October 20, 2015, http://www.moth-erjones.com/environment/2012/10/sugar-industry-lies-campaign.

22. Ibid.

23. William Joseph, "Giving His Addiction Up to God," *Guideposts*, accessed July 29, 2015, https:// www.guideposts.org/comfort-hope/health-well-being/ dealing-with-illness/addiction/giving-his-addiction-up-to-god?nopaging=1.

24. Ibid.

25. Ibid.

26. Alex, "The Psychology Behind Sugar Addictions."

Chapter 3
The Main Event: You Versus Sugar

1. "Sugar Consumption at a Crossroads," Credit Suisse Research and Analytics, (September 2013): 20, accessed August 15, 2015, https://doc.research-and-analytics.csfb.com/docView?language=ENG&source=u lg&format=PDF&document_id=1022457401&serialid= atRE31ByPkIjEXa%2fp3AyptOvIGdxTK833tLZ1E7Aw lQ%3d.

2. Walter Willett, "Ask the Expert: Controlling Your Weight," The Nutrition Source, accessed August 31, 2015, http://www.hsph.harvard.edu/nutritionsource/ weight-control/.

3. "History," The Nurses' Health Study, accessed August 31, 2015, http://www.channing.harvard.edu/nhs/?page_ id=70.

4. Steve Milano, "The Cholesterol Myth: Is Sugar the Big Culprit?" Preventive Cardiology Inc., June 18, 2014, accessed August 15, 2015, http://preventivecardiolo-gyinc.com/cholesterol-myth/.

5. P. W. Siri and R. M. Krauss, "Influence of Dietary Carbohydrate and Fat on LDL and HDL Particle Distributions," *Current Atherosclerosis Reports* 7, no. 6 (November 2005): 455–9, as referenced in Milano, "The Cholesterol Myth."

6. Milano, "The Cholesterol Myth"; see also Jean A. Welsh et al., "Caloric Sweetener Consumption and Dyslipidemia Among US Adults," *Journal of the American Medical Association* 303, no. 15 (2010): 1490–1497. doi:10.1001/jama.2010.449.

7. Salynn Boyles, "High-Sugar Diet Linked to Cholesterol," WebMD, April 20, 2010, accessed August 15, 2015, http://www.webmd.com/heart-disease/news/20100420/high-sugar-diet-linked-lower-good-cholesterol.

8. Mark Hyman, "Eggs Don't Cause Heart Attacks—Sugar Does," January 8, 2015, accessed August 15, 2015, http://drhyman.com/blog/2014/02/07/eggs-dont-cause-heart-attacks-sugar/.

9. Quanhe Yang et al., "Added Sugar Intake and Cardiovascular Diseases Mortality Among US Adults," *JAMA Internal Medicine* 174, no. 4 (2014):516–524. doi: 10.1001/jamainternmed.2013.13563, as referenced in Hyman, "Eggs Don't Cause Heart Attacks—Sugar Does."

10. Hyman, "Eggs Don't Cause Heart Attacks—Sugar Does."

11. Simin Liu et al., "A Prospective Study of Dietary Glycemic Load, Carbohydrate Intake, and Risk of Coronary Heart Disease in US Women," *American Journal of Clinical Nutrition* 71, no. 6 (June 2000): 1455–1461.

12. S. Basu et al., "The Relationship of Sugar to Population-Level Diabetes Prevalence: An Econometric Analysis of Repeated Cross-Sectional Data," *Public Library*

of Science One 8, no. 2 (2013): e57873. doi:10.1371/journal.pone.0057873.

13. As referenced in Laura Stevens, "The Sugar Wars: Using Diet to Treat ADHD Symptoms in Children," ADDitude, accessed October 20, 2015, http://www.additudemag.com/adhd/article/2861.html.

14. Ibid.

15. Tami Urbanek, "ADD and ADHD Symptoms Can Be a Sign of Excess Sugar and Boredom," Natural News, May 2, 2011, accessed August 15, 2015, http://www.naturalnews.com/032247_ADHD_sugar.html#ixzz3iv7Cqmb.

16. "Can Reducing Sugar Ease Autism Symptoms? Mouse Study Suggests It May," Autism Speaks, June 10, 2015, accessed August 15, 2015, https://www.autismspeaks.org/science/science-news/can-reducing-sugar-ease-autism-symptoms-mouse-study-suggests-it-may.

17. "Harmful Effects of Excess Sugar," Ask Dr. Sears, accessed August 15, 2015, http://www.askdrsears.com/topics/feeding-eating/family-nutrition/sugar/harmful-effects-excess-sugar.

18. Tammy Sutherland, "5 Foods That Will Destroy Your Teeth," Best Health, accessed August 15, 2015, www.besthealthmag.ca/best-you/oral-health/5-foods-that-will-destroy-your-teeth#06rFizC4IbaUFZtA.99.

19. Joseph Mercola, "Avoid Sugar to Help Slow Aging," Mercola.com, February 22, 2012, accessed October 20, 2015, http://articles.mercola.com/sites/articles/archive/2012/02/22/how-sugar-accelerates-aging.aspx; see also Joseph Mercola, "Sugar May Be Bad,

but This Sweetener Called Fructose Is Far More Deadly," Mercola.com, January 2, 2010, accessed August 15, 2015, http://articles.mercola.com/sites/articles/archive/2010/01/02/highfructose-corn-syrup-alters-human-metabolism.aspx.

20. Ibid.

21. Karyn Repinski, "Face Facts About Sugar: The Surprising Reason Eating Too Much Can Cause Wrinkles—And 5 Steps to Ensure That It Won't," *Prevention*, November 3, 2011, accessed August 16, 2015, http://www.prevention.com/beauty/natural-beauty/how-sugar-ages-your-skin.

22. Ibid.

23. Ibid.

24. Ibid.

25. G. L. Austin et al., "A Very Low-Carbohydrate Diet Improves Gastroesophageal Reflux and Its Symptoms," *Digestive Diseases and Sciences* 51, no. 8 (August 2006): 1307–12.

26. Amy Campbell, "Diabetes and GERD: Are They Linked? (Part 1)," Diabetes Self-Management, July 9, 2012, accessed October 20, 2015, http://www.diabetes-selfmanagement.com/blog/diabetes-and-gerd-are-they-linked-part-1/.

27. Jacqueline Jacques, "The Role of Your Thyroid in Metabolism and Weight Control," Obesity Action Coalition, accessed October 21, 2015, http://www.obesityaction.org/educational-resources/resource-articles-2/general-articles/

the-role-of-your-thyroid-in-metabolism-and-weight-control.

28. "What Is the Normal Range for Blood Sugar Levels, and What Blood Sugar Level Constitutes a True Emergency?" ABC News, August 14, 2008, accessed October 20, 2015, http://abcnews.go.com/Health/DiabetesScreening/story?id=3812946.

29. Cherie Calbom, "Sugar and Thyroid Blues: Do You Have Impaired Thyroid Function?" The Juice Lady, accessed October 20, 2015, http://www.juiceladycherie.com/Juice/sugar-thyroid-blues.

30. Patrick Quillin, "Cancer's Sweet Tooth," Nutrition Science News, April 2000, accessed October 20, 2015, http://www.mercola.com/article/sugar/sugar_cancer.htm.

31. "Food, Nutrition, Physical Activity, and the Prevention of Cancer," World Cancer Research Fund / American Institute for Cancer Research, 2007, accessed October 20, 2015, http://www.dietandcancerreport.org/cancer_resource_center/downloads/Second_Expert_Report_full.pdf; see also Taubes, "Is Sugar Toxic?"

32. Taubes, "Is Sugar Toxic?"

33. Ibid.

34. Cantley also simply said, "Sugar scares me." See Taubes, "Is Sugar Toxic?"

35. Taubes, "Is Sugar Toxic?"

36. Sarah Myhill, "Hypoglycaemia—The Full Story," updated April 1, 2015, accessed August 26, 2015,

http://www.drmyhill.co.uk/wiki/Hypoglycaemia_-_the_full_story.

37. Simin Liu et al., "A Prospective Study of Dietary Glycemic Load, Carbohydrate Intake, and Risk of Coronary Heart Disease in US Women," American Journal of Clinical Nutrition 71, no. 6 (June 2000): 1455–1461, as referenced in Barbara V. Howard and Judith Wylie-Rosett, "AHA Scientific Statement: Sugar and Cardiovascular Disease," Circulation 106 (2002): 523–527. doi:10.1161/01.CIR.0000019552.77778.04.

38. Talya Lavi et al., "The Acute Effect of Various Glycemic Index Dietary Carbohydrates on Endothelial Function in Nondiabetic Overweight and Obese Subjects," Journal of the American College of Cardiology 53, no. 24 (June 2009): 2283–2287. doi:10.1016/j.jacc.2009.03.025, as referenced in Clarence Bass, "More Evidence Every Meal Counts," Ripped, 2009, accessed October 20, 2015, http://www.cbass.com/Sugaryfoods_arteries.htm.

39. Ibid.

40. Yang et al., "Added Sugar Intake and Cardiovascular Disease Mortality Among US Adults"; see also Lawrence de Koning et al., "Sweetened Beverage Consumption, Incident Coronary Heart Disease, and Biomarkers of Risk in Men," Circulation 125, no. 14 (April 10, 2012): 1735–41. doi:10.1161/CIRCULATIONAHA.111.067017.

41. Marsha Nunley, "Sugar and Insomnia," Marsha Nunley, MD, December 23, 2011, accessed August 17, 2015,

https://marshanunleymd.wordpress.com/2011/12/23/
sugar-and-insomnia/.

42. Ibid.

Chapter 4
Knock Out Foggy Sugar Brain, Bad Mood, and Depression

1. Rahul Agrawal and Fernando Gomez-Pinilla, "'Metabolic Syndrome' in the Brain: Deficiency in Omega-3 Fatty Acid Exacerbates Dysfunctions in Insulin Receptor Signaling and Cognition," Journal of Physiology 590, Pt. 10 (May 15, 2012): 2485–2499. doi:10.1113/jphysiol.2012.230078.

2. Myhill, "Hypoglycaemia—The Full Story."

3. Lucia Kerti et al., "Higher Glucose Levels Associated with Lower Memory and Reduced Hippocampal Microstructure," Neurology 81, no. 20 (November 12, 2013): 1746–1752, http://dx.doi.org/10.1212/01.wnl. 0000435561.00234.ee.

4. Ibid.

5. Ronald M. Lawrence, "A Medical Doctors Report: A Report by Ronald M. Lawrence MD, PhD," Gero Vita International, accessed September 1, 2015, http://www. kats-korner.com/health/mdreport.html.

6. Nicole M. Avena, Pedro Rada, and Bartley G. Hoebel, "Evidence for Sugar Addiction: Behavioral and Neurochemical Effects of Intermittent, Excessive Sugar Intake," *Neuroscience and Biobehavioral*

   Reviews 32, no. 1 (2008): 20–39. doi:10.1016/j.neu-biorev.2007.04.019.

7. Roni Caryn Rabin, "Blood Sugar Control Linked to Memory Decline, Study Says," *New York Times*, December 31, 2008, accessed August 15, 2015, http://www.nytimes.com/2009/01/01/health/31memory.html?_r=0.

8. James E. Gangwisch et al., "High Glycemic Index Diet As a Risk Factor for Depression: Analyses from the Women's Health Initiative," *American Journal of Clinical Nutrition* (June 24, 2015). doi:10.3945/ajcn.114.103846.

9. "Junk Food May Increase Depression Risk," Columbia University Medical Center, July 29, 2015, accessed August 25, 2015, http://newsroom.cumc.columbia.edu/blog/2015/07/29/junk-food-may-increase-depression-risk/.

10. "Depression Link to Processed Food," BBC News, November 2, 2009, accessed August 16, 2015, http://news.bbc.co.uk/2/hi/health/8334353.stm.

11. A. N. Westover and L. B. Marangell, "A Cross-National Relationship between Sugar Consumption and Major Depression?" *Depression and Anxiety* 16, no. 3 (2002):118–20, accessed October 20, 2015, http://www.ncbi.nlm.nih.gov/pubmed/12415536?access_num=12415536&link_type=MED.

12. Scott Olson ND, "What Sugar Does to Your Brain," Wellsphere, November 12, 2008, accessed October 21,

2015, http://www.wellsphere.com/healthy-eating-article/
what-sugar-does-to-your-brain/490861.

13. "The Brain and Oxidative Stress," MitoQ, accessed
October 26, 2015, http://www.mitoq.com/mitoq-univer-
sity/the-brain-and-oxidative-stress/.

14. M. Peet, "International Variations in the Outcome of
Schizophrenia and the Prevalence of Depression in
Relation to National Dietary Practices: An Ecological
Analysis," *British Journal of Psychiatry* 184 (May
2004): 404–8, accessed August 16, 2015, http://www.
ncbi.nlm.nih.gov/pubmed/15123503.

15. Gregoire, "This Is What Sugar Does to Your Brain."

16. Ibid.

17. "Depression," Food for the Brain, accessed November 23,
2015, http://www.foodforthebrain.org/nutrition-solutions/
depression/about-depression.aspx.

18. Ibid.

19. Peet, "International Variations in the Outcome of
Schizophrenia."

20. R. Molteni et al., "A High-Fat, Refined Sugar Diet
Reduces Hippocampal Brain-Derived Neurotrophic
Factor, Neuronal Plasticity, and Learning," Neurosci-
ence 112, no. 4 (2002): 803–14.

21. Scott Olson ND, "What Sugar Does to Your Brain,"
OlsonND, accessed October 21, 2015, http://www.
olsonnd.com/what-sugar-does-to-your-brain/.

22. Peet, "International Variations in the Outcome of Schizophrenia," as referenced in Olson, "What Sugar Does to Your Brain."

23. Lawrence, "A Medical Doctors Report."

24. Katie Adolphus, Clare L. Lawton, and Louise Dye, "The Effects of Breakfast on Behavior and Academic Performance in Children and Adolescents," *Frontiers in Human Neuroscience* 7 (2013): 423. doi:10.3389/fnhum.2013.00425.

25. Lawrence, "A Medical Doctors Report."

26. Nyomi Graef, "Can Vitamin C Supplements Boost Mood, Memory, Intelligence and Brain Function?" Extra Happiness, January 10, 2011, accessed September 1, 2015, http://extrahappiness.com/happiness/?p=4415.

27. "Boron Osteoporosis, Osteopenia," Osteopenia and Osteoporosis Treatments and Cures, accessed September 1, 2015, http://www.osteopenia3.com/Boron-Osteoporosis.html.

Chapter 5
Diabetes, Hypoglycemia, and Blood Sugar Imbalances: Down for the Count

1. "What Is Normal Blood Sugar?" Diabetic Mediterranean Diet, accessed October 26, 2015, http://diabeticmediter-raneandiet.com/what-is-normal-blood-sugar/.

2. Centers for Disease Control and Prevention, "More Than 29 Million Americans Have Diabetes; 1 in 4 Doesn't

Know," news release, June 10, 2014, http://www.cdc.gov/media/releases/2014/p0610-diabetes-report.html.

3. Kristina Fiore, "Hypewatch: 100 Million Diabetic Americans in the Dark?" MedPage Today, November 19, 2014, accessed October 26, 2015, http://www.medpagetoday.com/Endocrinology/Diabetes/48712.

4. "Statistics About Diabetes," American Diabetes Association, last modified May 18, 2015, accessed October 26, 2015, http://www.diabetes.org/diabetes-basics/statistics/.

5. Centers for Disease Control and Prevention, "New Cases of Diagnosed Diabetes on the Rise," news release, October 30, 2008, http://www.cdc.gov/media/pressrel/2008/r081030.htm.

6. Centers for Disease Control and Prevention, Diabetes Report Card 2014, (Atlanta, Georgia: Centers for Disease Control and Prevention, 2015), accessed October 26, 2015, http://www.cdc.gov/diabetes/pdfs/library/diabetesreportcard2014.pdf.

7. Lisa Nainggolan, "Incidence of Diabetes in US Doubles in 30 Years," Medscape, June 21, 2006, accessed November 20, 2015, http://www.medscape.com/viewarticle/788547.

8. Taubes, "Is Sugar Toxic?"http://www.nytimes.com/2011/04/17/magazine/mag-17Sugar-t.html?_r=0

9. Ibid.

10. Ibid.

11. Ibid.

12. Ibid.

13. Ibid.

14. Ibid.

15. Scott M. Grundy, "Metabolic Syndrome Pandemic," *Arteriosclerosis, Thrombosis, and Vascular Biology* 28 (2008): 629–636. doi:10.1161; "Insulin Resistance and Prediabetes," National Institute of Diabetes and Digestive and Kidney Diseases, accessed November 23, 2015, http://www.niddk.nih.gov/health-information/health-topics/Diabetes/insulin-resistance-prediabetes/Pages/index.aspx.

16. Mirella Hage, Mira S. Zantout, and Sami T. Azar, "Thyroid Disorders and Diabetes Mellitus," Journal of Thyroid Research 2011 (2011), http://dx.doi.org/10.4061/2011/439463.

17. Taubes, "Is Sugar Toxic?" http://www.nytimes.com/2011/04/17/magazine/mag-17Sugar-t.html?_r=0

18. Ibid.

19. Ibid.

20. Loszach Report, "Killing Us Sweetly," The Loszach Blog, August 8, 2012, accessed August 2, 2015, https://loszachreport.wordpress.com/2012/08/08/killing-us-sweetly/.

21. Taubes, "Is Sugar Toxic?" http://www.nytimes.com/2011/04/17/magazine/mag-17Sugar-t.html?_r=0

22. Ibid.

23. Kristen L. Knutson, "Impact of Sleep and Sleep Loss on Glucose Homeostasis and Appetite Regulation," *Journal*

of Clinical Sleep Medicine 2, no. 2 (June 2007): 187–197. doi:10.1016/j.jsmc.2007.03.004.

24. Eve Van Cauter et al., "The Impact of Sleep Deprivation on Hormones and Metabolism," *Medscape Neurology* 7, no. 1 (2005), accessed June 23, 2015, http://www.medscape.org/viewarticle/502825.

Chapter 6
Taking Off the Gloves: How to Strengthen Your Immune System

1. New Scientist 23 Nov 1991, pg 13 http://www.academia.edu/3816684/All_about_Splenda October 27, 2015

2. Kim Painter, "Does a Spoonful of Sugar Help the Flu Take Hold?" USA TODAY, October 5, 2009, accessed August 1, 2015, http://usatoday30.usatoday.com/news/health/painter/2009-10-04-your-health_N.htm.

3. Albert Sanchez et al., "Role of Sugars in Human Neutrophilic Phagocytosis," *The American Journal of Clinical Nutrition* 26 (November 1973): 1180–1184.

4. Tatfeng Y. Mirabeau and Enitan S. Samson, "Effect of Allium Cepa and Allium Sativum on Some Immunological Cells in Rats," *African Journal of Traditional, Complementary, and Alternative Medicines* 9, no. 3 (2012): 374–379.

5. Quillin, "Cancer's Sweet Tooth."

6. Tara Parker-Pope, "The Science of Chicken Soup," *New York Times*, October 12, 2007, accessed August 2,

2015, http://well.blogs.nytimes.com/2007/10/12/the-science-of-chicken-soup/.

7. D. A. Hughes et al., "The Effect of Beta-Carotene Supplementation on the Immune Function of Blood Monocytes from Healthy Male Nonsmokers," *The Journal of Laboratory and Clinical Medicine* 129, no. 3 (March 1997): 307–319.

8. Recipe can be found at Alexandra Du Toit, "Master Tonic: Ingredients and Directions," Earthie Mama, accessed August 2, 2015, http://www.earthiemama.com/master-tonic.html.

Chapter 7
Sucker Punch the Extra Weight

1. Ben Greenfield, "How Sugar Makes You Fat," Greenfield Fitness Systems, accessed October 21, 2015, https://greenfieldfitnesssystems.com/article-archive/how-sugar-makes-you-fat/.

2. K. A. Page et al., "Effects of Fructose vs Glucose on Regional Cerebral Blood Flow in Brain Regions Involved with Appetite and Reward Pathways," *JAMA* 309, no. 1 (January 2, 2013): 63–70. doi:10.1001/jama.2012.116975.

3. Mercola, "Avoid Sugar to Help Slow Aging."

4. "Do Sports Drinks Affect Your Teeth?" Oxley Park Dental Practice, accessed October 27, 2015, http://www.oxleyparkdentalpractice.co.uk/2014/10/do-sports-drinks-affect-your-teeth/.

5. "Hay Diet," Diet.com, accessed October 28, 2015, http://www.diet.com/g/hay-diet.

6. James Khan, "Does Maintaining Acid Alkaline Balance Benefit Your Health?" DetoxifyNow.com, accessed October 28, 2015, http://detoxifynow.com/acid-alkaline-balance-review/.

7. S. T. Reddy et al., "Effect of Low-Carbohydrate High-Protein Diets on Acid-Base Balance, Stone-Forming Propensity, and Calcium Metabolism," *American Journal of Kidney Diseases* 40, no. 2 (August 2002): 265–74, as referenced in Candace McNaughton, "The Acid Alkaline Balance," Sound Consumer, October 2009, http://www.pccnaturalmarkets.com/sc/0910/sc0910-acid-alkaline.html.

8. Sang Whang, *Reverse Aging* (Miami, FL: JSP Publishing, 2001).

9. O. A. Jones, M. L. Maguire, and J. L. Griffin, "Environmental Pollution and Diabetes: a Neglected Association," *Lancet* 371, no. 9609 (January 26, 2008): 287–8. doi:10.1016/S0140-6736(08)60147-6.

10. I. A. Lang et al., "Association of Urinary Bisphenol A Concentration with Medical Disorders and Laboratory Abnormalities in Adults," *JAMA* 300, no. 11 (September 17, 2008): 1303–10. doi:10.1001/jama.300.11.1303.

11. "Study Finds Industrial Pollution Begins in the Womb," Environmental Working Group, accessed October 21, 2015, http://www.ewg.org/kid-safe-chemicals-act-blog/ewg-research/; see also Mark Hyman, "How Toxins

Make You Fat: 4 Steps to Get Rid of Toxic Weight," October 18, 2014, accessed October 21, 2015, http://drhyman.com/blog/2012/02/20/how-toxins-make-you-fat-4-steps-to-get-rid-of-toxic-weight/.

12. Holly, "Sugar Addiction, Detox and Gaining Control Over Food," *300 Pounds Down Blog*, June 7, 2013, http://www.300poundsdown.com/2013/06/sugar-addic-tion-detox-and-gaining-control-over-food.html.

Chapter 8
The Sugar Shopping Guide

1. "How to Spot Sugar on Food Labels," Hungry for Change, accessed July 31, 2015, http://www.hungry-forchange.tv/article/how-to-spot-sugar-on-food-labels, accessed July 31, 2015.

2. Katherine L. Tucker et al., "Colas, but Not Other Car-bonated Beverages, Are Associated with Low Bone Mineral Density in Older Women: The Framingham Osteoporosis Study," *The American Journal of Clinical Nutrition* 84 (2006): 936–42; see also "Sugar Pro-duces Bitter Results for the Environment," Earth Talk, accessed July 28, 2015, http://environment.about.com/od/pollution/a/sugar.htm.

3. Taubes, "Is Sugar Toxic?"

4. "Much High Fructose Corn Syrup Contaminated with Mercury, New Study Finds," Institute for Agricul-ture and Trade Policy, January 26, 2009, accessed September 2, 2015, http://www.iatp.org/documents/

much-high-fructose-corn-syrup-contaminated-with-mercury-new-study-finds.

5. Richard R. Johnson et al., "Sugar, Uric Acid, and the Etiology of Diabetes and Obesity," *Diabetes* 62, no. 10 (October 2013): 3307–3315. doi:10.2337/db12-1814.

6. Harvard, "Abundance of Fructose Not Good for the Liver, Heart."

7. American Chemical Society, "Soda Warning? High-Fructose Corn Syrup Linked to Diabetes, New Study Suggests," ScienceDaily, accessed September 2, 2015, http://www.sciencedaily.com/releases/2007/08/070823094819.htm.

8. Robert Lustig, "Fructose: the Poison Index," *The Guardian*, October 21, 2013, accessed July 28, 2015, http://www.theguardian.com/commentisfree/2013/oct/21/fructose-poison-sugar-industry-pseudoscience.

9. Ibid.

10. Xiaosen Ouyang et al., "Fructose Consumption as a Risk Factor for Non-Alcoholic Fatty Liver Disease," *Journal of Hepatology* 48, no. 6 (June 2008): 993–999. doi:http://dx.doi.org/10.1016/j.jhep.2008.02.011, as referenced in Sarah Cimperman, "The Health Hazards of Agave and Fructose," Wisdom, accessed June 8, 2011, http://wisdom-magazine.com/Article.aspx/1838.

11. Manal F. Abdelmaled et al., "Increased Fructose Consumption Is Associated with Fibrosis Severity in Patients with Nonalcoholic Fatty Liver Disease," *Hepatology* 51, no. 6 (June 2010): 1961–1971. doi: 10.1002/

hep.23535, as referenced in Cimperman, "The Health Hazards of Agave and Fructose."

12. Joseph Mercola, "Aspartame Update: Coke Illegally Claims Diet Soda Can Combat Obesity, and Researchers Propose Autism Link," Mercola.com, July 22, 2015, accessed August 9, 2015, http://articles.mercola.com/sites/articles/archive/2015/07/22/aspartame-diet-soda-autism-link.aspx.

13. Joseph Mercola, "How Artificial Sweeteners Confuse Your Body into Storing Fat and Inducing Diabetes," Mercola.com, December 23, 2014, accessed August 9, 2015, http://articles.mercola.com/sites/articles/archive/2014/12/23/artificial-sweeteners-confuse-body.aspx.

14. Shawn, "Sugar Twin: That Stuff Will Kill You," *Confessions of a Changed Shawn Blog*, May 5, 2011, accessed August 9, 2015, https://realfph.wordpress.com/2011/05/05/sugar-twin-that-stuff-will-kill-you/.

15. S. S. Schiffman and K. I. Rother, "Sucralose, a Synthetic Organochlorine Sweetener: Overview of Biological Issues," *Journal of Toxicology and Environmental Health* Part B 16, no. 7 (2013): 399–451. doi:10.1080/10937404.2013.842523, as referenced in Jessica Girdwain, "Is Splenda Really Safe?" *Prevention*, December 17, 2013, accessed September 2, 2015, http://www.prevention.com/food/healthy-eating-tips/health-risks-sucralose.

16. Ibid.

17. Ibid.

18. Joseph Mercola, "Aspartame: Could This Headache Causing Neurotoxin Be On Its Way Out?" Mercola.com, May 14, 2015, accessed August 9, 2015, http://articles. mercola.com/sites/articles/archive/2015/05/14/artificial-sweeteners-diet-soda.aspx.

19. Ibid.

20. Ibid.

21. Andrew Schneider, "Asian Honey, Banned in Europe, Is Flooding US Grocery Shelves," Food Safety News, August 15, 2011, http://www.foodsafetynews. com/2011/08/honey-laundering/#.VieYJulq3IU; see also Andrew Schneider, "Tests Show Most Store Honey Isn't Honey," Food Safety News, November 7, 2011, accessed August 9, 2015, http://www.foodsafetynews. com/2011/11/tests-show-most-store-honey-isnt-honey/#. Vee.

22. Schneider, "Asian Honey, Banned in Europe, Is Flooding US Grocery Shelves."

23. Earth Talk, "Where Have All the Honeybees Gone?" *E/The Environmental Magazine* 15, no, 23 (June 7–13, 2007); see also Earth Talk, "Why Are Honeybees Disappearing?" About News, accessed October 21, 2015, http://environment.about.com/od/biodiversityconservation/a/honeybees.htm.

24. Ibid.

25. Ibid.

26. Christopher A. Mullin et al., "High Levels of Miticides and Agrochemicals in North American Apiaries: Implications for Honey Bee Health," *Public Library*

of Science-One 5, no, 3 (2010): e9754. doi:10.1371/journal.pone.0009754, as referenced in Ned Potter, "Honeybees Dying: Scientists Wonder Why, and Worry About Food Supply," ABC News, March 25, 2010, accessed June 6, 2015, http://abcnews.go.com/Technology/honey-bees-dying-scientists-suspect-pesticides-disease-worry/story?id=10191391.

27. Organic Consumers Association, as referenced in Earth Talk, "Where Have All the Honeybees Gone?"

28. Earth Talk, "Where Have All the Honeybees Gone?"

29. Ibid.

30. Alexei Barrionuevo, "Honeybees Vanish, Leaving Keepers in Peril," *New York Times*, February 27, 2007, accessed June 6, 2015, http://www.nytimes.com/2007/02/27/business/27bees.html?pagewanted=1&_r=0.

31. Potter, "Honeybees Dying."

Chapter 9
The Ten-Step Sugar Detox Plan:
How to Force Sugar to Throw in the Towel

1. "Insulin Resistance," Diabetes.co.uk, accessed August 24, 2015, http://www.diabetes.co.uk/insulin-resistance.html.

2. Ezra Fieser, "Organic Coffee: Why Latin America's Farmers Are Abandoning It," *The Christian Science Monitor*, December 29, 2009, http://www.csmonitor.com/World/Americas/2010/0103/

Organic-coffee-Why-Latin-America-s-farmers-are-abandoning-it.

3. Joseph Mercola, "If You Drink Coffee Make Sure It Is Organic," Mercola.com, January 30, 2010, accessed August 25, 2015, http://articles.mercola.com/sites/articles/archive/2010/01/30/if-you-drink-coffee-make-sure-it-is-organic.aspx.

4. Brent A. Bauer, "What Is Wheatgrass, and Should I Add It to My Smoothies for Better Health?" Mayo Clinic, January 22, 2014, http://www.mayoclinic.org/healthy-living/nutrition-and-healthy-eating/expert-answers/wheatgrass/faq-20058018.

5. Arlet V. Nedeltcheva et al., "Sleep Curtailment Is Accompanied by Increased Intake of Calories from Snacks," *American Journal of Clinical Nutrition* 89, no. 1 (January 2009): 126–133. doi:10.3945/ajcn.2008.26574, as referenced in Amy Paturel, "Sleep More, Weigh Less," WebMD, June 30, 2014, http://www.webmd.com/diet/sleep-and-weight-loss?page=1.

6. Paturel, "Sleep More, Weigh Less."

7. Craig Lambert, "Deep into Sleep," *Harvard Magazine*, July-August 2005, accessed August 24, 2015, http://harvardmagazine.com/2005/07/deep-into-sleep.html.

8. Sharon V. Thompson, Donna M. Winham, and Andrea M. Hutchins, "Bean and Rice Meals Reduce Postprandial Glycemic Response in Adults with Type 2 Diabetes: a Cross-Over Study," *Nutrition Journal* 11 (2012): 23. doi:10.1186/1475-2891-11-23.

9. Dr. Joel Fuhrman, "Dr. Fuhrman's 3-Day Sugar Detox," Doctor Oz.com, October 9, 2014, accessed August 26, 2015, http://www.doctoroz.com/article/dr-fuhrmans-3-day-sugar-detox?page=3.

10. Ibid.

CONNECT WITH US!

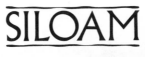
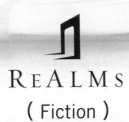

Ignite Your SPIRITUAL HEALTH

with these FREE Newsletters

CHARISMA HEALTH
Get information and news on health-related topics and studies, and tips for healthy living.

POWER UP! FOR WOMEN
Receive encouraging teachings that will empower you for a Spirit-filled life.

CHARISMA MAGAZINE NEWSLETTER
Get top-trending articles, Christian teachings, entertainment reviews, videos and more.

CHARISMA NEWS WEEKLY
Get the latest breaking news from an evangelical perspective every Monday.

SIGN UP AT:
nl.charismamag.com

CHARISMA MEDIA